DIET AND THE DISEASE
OF CIVILIZATION

DIET AND THE DISEASE OF CIVILIZATION

ADRIENNE ROSE BITAR

RUTGERS UNIVERSITY PRESS

New Brunswick, Camden, and Newark, New Jersey, and London

Library of Congress Cataloging-in-Publication Data

Names: Bitar, Adrienne Rose, 1986– author.
Title: Diet and the disease of civilization / Adrienne Rose Bitar.
Description: New Brunswick, New Jersey : Rutgers University Press, [2017] |
  Includes bibliographical references and index.
Identifiers: LCCN 2017014959 (print) | LCCN 2017019969 (ebook) | ISBN
  9780813589664 (E-pub) | ISBN 9780813589688 (Web PDF) | ISBN 9780813589657
  (cloth : alk. paper) | ISBN 9780813589640 (pbk. : alk. paper)
Subjects: LCSH: Diet. | Nutrition—Social aspects.
Classification: LCC RA784 (ebook) | LCC RA784 .B546 2017 (print) | DDC
  613.2—dc23
LC record available at https://lccn.loc.gov/2017014959

A British Cataloging-in-Publication record for this book is available from the British Library.

www.rutgersuniversitypress.org

Manufactured in the United States of America

For my father and editor, Michael McIntyre Johnson

CONTENTS

DIET AND THE DISEASE
OF CIVILIZATION

INTRODUCTION

Diet books are some of the bestselling books of the twentieth century. By some accounts, the Atkins series has sold more than twenty million copies. *The South Beach Diet* sold about ten million and *Eat Right 4 Your Type* adds in another seven million. Combined, just these three diet books could fill every shelf in the Library of Congress and still have a copy left over to circulate at every American public library.

Obesity rates and the long, complicated history of food and diet explain a lot about why forty-five million Americans diet every year and weight loss is an estimated $60-billion industry.[1] As oft-cited statistics indicate, obesity rates have more than doubled in the last generation, growing from just under 15 percent in the 1960s to 35 percent today.[2] Morbid obesity rates quadrupled between 1986 and 2000.[3] Today, two out of every three Americans are overweight or obese. In 1997, the surgeon general declared a "war on obesity," calling it an epidemic which endangered the very future of the nation. By 2002, another surgeon general called obesity "the 'terror within', a threat that is every bit as real to America as weapons of mass destruction."[4]

Diet books do more than offer insight into statistics like these. With the onset of the obesity epidemic about thirty years ago, the books became myths and manifestos, with broader concerns and higher stakes. They now look more like manuals to make the world a better place. Like other powerful narratives, diet books offer insight into how America sees itself, blames itself, and what kind of civilization it promises to make for itself.

The scholar R.W.B. Lewis once explained that the history of a culture is a dialogue, a sometimes bruising contact of opposites that uses specifics to stand in for larger, more powerful ideas. Diets, like all good cultural touchstones, stand in for the bigger debate about history, salvation, nature, money, power, sin, hope, innocence, experience, time, and all the other ideas that make the world worth thinking about. And Lewis writes that a scholar's work is not to settle the terms of the discussion—to judge right and wrong, declare a victor—but to divine the "images and 'story' that animate the ideas and are their imaginative and usually more compelling equivalent."[5] Diet books enclose these big ideas to reveal, in Lewis's words, "a certain habitual story" that gets repeated endlessly, from one decade to the next, from one generation to the next, a story about a fallen civilization that might just still do right.

Diets retell the narrative backbone for our national consciousness: a tragedy of the jeremiad lamenting a lost Eden, simmering with potential, and always grasping for a better world. It is unsurprising that diets narrate what is, arguably, the most familiar literary narrative in the Western world. More important for a deeper understanding, however, is how these diets use the banal, often boring material of breakfast-lunch-dinner and the quest for self-improvement to channel larger concerns about the success or failure of America.

It is easy to confuse American dieting and diet books. The diet itself—the breakfast-lunch-dinner plan—is often the least interesting part of the diet book. Of the four hundred diet books surveyed for this study, the practical details of the diet take up on average less than 20 percent of the total content. Recipes and nutrition tables are minor compared to the pages devoted to dieter testimonials, autobiographical reflection, and food philosophies. Usually the actual advice can be summarized in a few words: either eat grains and cut meat or eat meat and cut grains. Exercise. Don't overdo it on sweets. Some mono-diets promote a single food or dish: juice, bananas, or cabbage soup. Others promote whole cuisines, like the

Mediterranean diet. Still others couch themselves as medical or spiritual or religious. But these are mere details when compared with the *stories* told by diet books—stories that have captivated tens of millions of readers over the last hundred years.

By a rough count, *Diet and the Disease of Civilization* draws from four hundred diet books published over the last hundred years. An original archive was composed from hundreds of these books—ebooks and pamphlets and promotional materials, every diet book at dozens of Goodwills, and ephemera such as grocery receipts, recipes, and food diaries. A Craigslist want ad led to the acquisition of a private collection: hundreds of food diaries, inspiration cards, carbohydrate counters, and diet books collected by one woman over the course of her lifetime. She bookmarked in a half dozen "before" photos in the diaries and never an "after"; often these personal things offer the greatest insight into the tender project of reading a diet book.

Before the 1990s, weight loss diets were usually categorized into two groups: "faddish" feminine diets and more "serious" medical advice. With the onset of the obesity epidemic, however, diet books began to look more like clarion calls for serious political and cultural reform. Weight loss suddenly became an American concern, with the health of the nation at risk. And diet books published in the last twenty years represent the first time the efforts of countercultural food activism, government health-promotion policy, federal food guidelines, and faddish weight loss diets have come together to truly create a unifying narrative of American health and disease.

This distinction, though arbitrary, may have distracted scholars from the significant shift in diet literature published since the onset of the obesity epidemic, roughly in the early 1990s. Scholarship has lagged on the topic. By taking a top-down approach, American perspectives on food often consider diet as a project of nation-building promoted by the federal government through initiatives like Michelle Obama's Let's Move program. A host of geopolitical, environmental, labor, human rights, and economic concerns also stress the global food system and occupy scholars working on these urgent issues. In terms of diet for weight loss, many discussions today still see diet as an individual concern, usually particular to overweight women. Though these themes are no doubt important, they have misled scholars into upholding that same arbitrary dichotomy between the serious and the silly in diet advice. The arbitrariness of this distinction explains volumes about how scholars and cultural critics have overlooked some of the best-selling books of the twentieth century.

A study of the American diet would raise these important and timely concerns. Yet this book is not that study because diet books are books of their own breed—they are stories that read a lot like scripts, laid out in text and fleshed out in the daily life of the dieter. They are useful fictions that function in the real world. Few academics have looked at diet books and no literary scholar has analyzed the role of these texts in shaping the stories American culture tells about its past and its future. Diet books, to borrow from Clifford Geertz, are the stories we tell ourselves about ourselves. And this book is a study of a people and their stories.

Diet and the Disease of Civilization follows a chronology of imaginary human origins. Four chapters analyze four diets—the Paleo diet, the Eden diet, the precolonial diet, and the detox diet—all of which follow the same familiar narrative. Along the arc of the Fall of Man, these diets remember an original, innocent world and mourn the descent of the human race into modern disease. This survey of just over four hundred diet books published since the 1910s reveals four locations of human origins and health: in the cave (the Paleo diet), the Garden of Eden (the Eden, or biblical, diet), the precolonial paradise (Pacific Island, or primitive, diet), and the preindustrial world (detox diet).

Chapter 1 maps out the Paleolithic diet. Paleo dieters today number into the millions and the diet—modeled loosely after ideas of Paleolithic nutrition and ways of life—has been called the defining diet of the early 2010s. Paleolithic diets belong to the long Western tradition of venerating preagricultural diets. Dieters believe that civilization has outpaced evolution and created a world hostile to human biology. Usually, utopian myths about food celebrate cornucopias of lavish, never-ending feasts but the Paleo myth redefines a new type of refined, slow pleasure. A peaceful vision of gender relations between cavemen and cavewomen—"cavepeople," maybe—who hunted, gathered, and lived in sexual harmony also overturns scholarly thinking about brutish cavemen masculinity.

Chapter 2 shifts away from evolutionary accounts of human history to a biblical understanding of genesis with Eden diets. Most historians today agree that contemporary weight loss diets are heirs of Puritan asceticism and long traditions of female fasting. Beauty ideals, they believe, have also grown out of the secularization of Christian suffering. However, Eden diets disavow suffering and redefine a special kind of pleasure, nuancing the relationship between the body and divine instincts. Eden diets promise a beautiful, blessed deliciousness that uses holy food to revive God-given instinct in a still-sacred human body created by God and handed down to Adam and all of humankind.

Chapter 3 moves from the Garden of Eden to an Edenic garden in a precolonial paradise. Precontact or primitive diets are based on the moment of colonial encounter in which a previously healthy race is brought into the modern world, introduced to contemporary foods, and subjected to the diseases of civilization. Unlike Paleo and Eden diets, primitive diets revive the old and sometimes ugly debate about race and human origins. These diets question whether human beings share a common ancestor or have such different origins as to require evolutionarily-specific diets. The diets refine the nostalgic "noble savage" theme by citing primitive disease as proof of a failed experiment. A foreboding darkens the dying savage story, suggesting the first to fall will not be the last and Westerners might soon follow in their fatal wake.

From precolonial paradises, the diets move to a world before industrialization. Chapter 4 considers detoxification diets. Detox diets, as they are more often called, maintain that environmental toxins have caused a host of modern diseases, everything from obesity to epilepsy and Alzheimer's. Detox diets look back to a preindustrial world, viewing toxins as a symbol for the hazards of modernity. Beginning in the late 1980s, detoxification diets helped introduce the metaphor of toxicity into food politics and politicized food and diet in a way that laid the foundation for today's alternative food movement. Detox's concept of the "toxic food environment" was later picked up by obesity prevention researchers and activists to explain food addiction. These diets demonstrate the porousness of the boundary between body and environment, revealing new ways that Americans have conceptualized the health effects of modern living and the postindustrial environment. And these diets reveal how Americans have interpreted the biological dangers of modernity in late twentieth-century medicine and culture.

Scholars have called the United States the most diet-conscious society on the planet.[6] Agricultural abundance, cultural diversity, the rapid pace of technological change, and an emphasis on free will all combined to create a nation which has constantly questioned the rights and wrongs of a national cuisine. Food creates categories of political and social identity—inside and out, us and them—that has particular relevance in a society that invests so much power in an individual's self-determination. If every forkful is a choice, then perhaps food is the best everyday expression of free will which, as sociologist E. Melanie DuPuis recently put it, speaks to basic tenets of the "Western idea of democracy and freedom."[7]

Choosing what to eat is difficult in a society characterized by constant innovation: new foods, new crops, new dishes, new restaurants, and new methods of preservation and food processing have created a dizzying glut of choices available to the American consumer. The average 2017 American supermarket carries about 40,000 unique items.[8] When Andy Warhol first painted *Campbell's Soup Cans* in 1962, he accurately represented Campbell's 32 varieties of soup. Today, Campbell's sells 272 different soup varieties: Cream of Bacon was the most recent addition to their condensed soup line.

New World abundance also changed culinary history forever. Called the Columbian Exchange, the fifteenth- and sixteenth-century transfer of plants and animals between the New World and the Old revolutionized global agriculture, diet, and cuisine. Tomatoes, peanuts, potatoes, cacao, chili peppers, and vanilla were all new to Europeans. Observers marveled at the array and availability of so many current staples of the global diet. As historian Hasia Diner notes, dreams of New World abundance were powerful currency in attracting hungry immigrants to a country "full of all sorts of excellent viands," as a 1605 play described the young British colony of Virginia.[9]

With so many excellent viands to choose from and the freedom to choose heavily freighted with ideas of freedom, it is no wonder that diet advice has been such a rich arena for larger debates about the American character. Most visibly, through regulations and guidelines, government officials have long issued top-down guidance about a healthy diet. Religious reformers, food activists, and medical experts have contributed competing narratives. More stealthily, diet book authors have written stories explaining what and how and why to eat in the United States. Taken as a whole, diet books provide the narrative key to understanding how all these sources combine to change definitions of proper diet and create a contested and complex system of moral evaluation and national identity.

Scholars generally cite William Banting's 1863 bestselling *Letter on Corpulence, Addressed to the Public* as the first diet plan.[10] Autobiographical and compassionate, the British undertaker chronicled his "obnoxious boils" and other physical ailments alongside the emotional pain of being a fat man in London, subject to cruel sneers and taunts. In consultation with his doctor, William Harvey, Banting lost over thirty-five pounds on a high-protein diet of meats, stale toast, and cooked fruits. His sixteen-page pamphlet quickly became a bestseller in both the United Kingdom and the United States. *Letter on Corpulence* went through twelve editions by 1900, selling between sixty and seventy thousand copies by 1878.[11] Banting's plan established two principles of the modern diet: that obesity is a physiological disease and "corpulence is a condition of the modern, Western age."[12] Other British diets followed suit, such as the 1883 *Advice to Stout People* or 1889 *Foods for the Fat*.[13]

Stateside, no single-authored book stands out. Respectable publications like *Scientific American* referred to Banting and London journals to prescribe tea, seaweed, sparkling red wine, and "tight lacing," or the British practice of lacing a man into a tight women's corset, to cure corpulence.[14] In fact, American weight loss advice at the end of the nineteenth century was chaotic, an entrepreneurial mix of sanitariums, hucksters, quacks, weight reducing devices, and patent medicines. In the late 1890s, Horace Fletcher, or "The Great Masticator," cultivated a wildly popular diet doctrine fixed on rigorous chewing. Even celebrities such as John D. Rockefeller and Upton Sinclair adhered to the plan to chew each bite of food thirty-two times (one chew for each tooth) for greater health and longevity.[15]

Earlier, beginning in the 1830s, a new religious health reform movement offered diet advice as part of the unified quest for physical and spiritual perfection, not weight loss. Reformers back then linked sexual health to spiritual purity and believed a flavorless, vegetarian diet would dampen sexual desire, mute the various appetites, and improve spiritual health. Reformers also pioneered a new self-help, can-do concept that Americans didn't need to accept disease and death as simply God's will. Instead, Americans could follow specific diets and ways of living to improve their well-being on earth.[16] Sylvester Graham (1794–1851), Presbyterian minister and Graham cracker namesake, led the crusade for strict vegetarianism in the 1830s, believing that meat excited the sexual appetite and decimated moral and bodily health.[17] For Graham, bread and bland foods "signified domestic order, civic health, and moral well-being." For Graham and his followers, American-grown wheat and wholesome, unseasoned bread would help "ensure America's place in the pantheon of civilized nations."[18]

Like Graham, John Harvey Kellogg (1852–1943) also prescribed a bland, vegetarian diet to reduce sexual activity and purify the spirit. An influential Seventh-Day Adventist better known today for his cereals, Kellogg was famous in his own time for his bizarre health treatments for the sickly rich: yogurt enemas, regulated sunbaths, and electric vibration treatments were administered at a posh 1,200-room sanitarium that treated celebrated patients such as Warren G. Harding, Thomas Edison, and Sojourner Truth.[19] Kellogg was also one of the first to incorporate scientific evaluations of calorific value into a prescriptive diet, using U.S. Department of Agriculture (USDA) composition tables in his 1908 Battle Creek Sanitarium System.[20]

At the end of the nineteenth century, chemist Wilbur Atwater served as the first director of research for the USDA. In 1894, he published the first composition table of food values. Distributed in a *Farmer's Bulletin* pamphlet, the table broke down common foods such as cauliflower or cod into the now-familiar categories of calories, protein, fat, and carbohydrate matter.[21] In analyzing foods by component, Atwater institutionalized the process by which diet attributes value to foods and organizes foods according to these evaluations. Like any system of organization, dietary evaluations invest previously mute objects with the capacity to symbolize some abstraction: a carrot, for example, stands in for vitamin A or a lamb shank represents protein. Atwater's work established methods to analyze food values that later proved indispensable to nutritional advice domestically and food relief efforts abroad.

Despite the diversity and fervor of food reformers, the American diet was not truly an urgent topic of national importance until World War I. The USDA released its first food guidelines, "Food for Young Children," in 1916, just as President Woodrow Wilson was turning his attention to food aid.[22] Under Wilson, Herbert Hoover headed the U.S. Food Administration (USFA), established in 1917 to provide food relief programs to Europe.[23] Massive food conservation efforts taught Americans about the ethical and health implications of certain foodstuffs—primarily meat, wheat, and sugar. At the same time, scientists discovered vitamins and "vitamania" swept the land, inspiring Americans with miracle cures and building the now multi-billion-dollar vitamin and supplement industry.[24]

Between 1914 and 1924, Hoover distributed about four million tons of food to Europe through USFA and the American Relief Association. Humanitarian ideals no doubt motivated the Wilson administration to prevent starvation in Europe, but Hoover also acknowledged the considerable aid could "stem the tide of Bolshevism" among Europe's hungry citizens.[25] The efforts earned him the nickname the Great Humanitarian; some historians now believe Hoover saved more lives than any other man in history due to his emergency relief efforts both in World War I Belgium and, later, during the devastating 1921–1923 famine in Soviet Russia.

Even with the far-reaching powers granted by the Lever Act of 1917 to requisition food, punish hoarders, ration staples, and set prices, Hoover publicly chose to invoke the spirit of patriotism to persuade Americans to voluntarily conserve food. Most obviously, the USFA instructed Americans to increase consumption of perishable fresh fruits and vegetables and reduce meat, wheat, and sugar. Nonperishable, high-calorie foods were shipped abroad. Hoover drew from Atwater's USDA nutrient and calorie measures to calculate which foods would best feed soldiers and famished Europeans. As Helen Zoe Veit recently noted, more than fourteen million Americans "'joined' the Food Administration by signing membership cards pledging themselves and their families to comply with food conservation measures."[26] "Righteous physical self-control" both confirmed patriotic sacrifice and allowed Americans (particularly women) to "demonstrate their mastery over their own bodies."[27]

Perhaps because Hoover chose not to ration, the language of health was third to moral virtue and patriotism in American diet discourse during World War I. Books such as the 1917 *War-Time Cook and Health Book* advised Americans on the healthfulness of low-calorie choices.[28] The frontispiece, reprinted from the Department of Food Conservation, explains "How You Can Serve Your Country" by doubling the use of greenstuffs to increase health *and* serve the nation.

Patriotism was also invoked in the fight against fat. Not only did fat people hoard calories, fat men couldn't fight. In 1914, journalist Vance Thompson introduced the diet book *Eat and Grow Thin: The Mahdah Menus* with the ominous story of how the "mighty French empire [fell] to pieces in the hands of a fat Napoleon." After the paunchy Napoleon doomed his nation, Thompson explained that "fat generation followed fat generation in a procession, at once tragic and grotesque, over the quaking earth." Fat was not only ugly but also made men weak, ridiculous, and, borrowing Thompson's words, foolish, grotesque, elephant-footed, and tragic. *Eat and Grow Thin* suggests a more broadly Western understanding of food during wartime, reflecting back on Napoleon's obese demise to raise the stakes on Western fatness to indicate the decline of Western civilization during the crisis of World War I.[29]

Dr. Lulu Hunt Peters's 1918 *Diet and Health, with Key to the Calories* most closely resembles a contemporary diet book. Unlike Thompson's damning approach to the hideous "tragedy in suet" that was a fat person's life, Peters was resolutely American in her simple menus of beefsteak and buttermilk and compassionate in her can-do attitude. Also unlike the Food Administration's conservation propaganda, *Diet and Health* was undeniably an aesthetic diet, giving tips for a graceful bearing and a beautiful complexion. Today Peters is called "America's first successful weight-loss guru," most likely because she used equal parts nutritional ethos and autobiographical pathos to translate nutritional data into easy-to-understand language.[30] Describing her own "long, long battle" with the "too, too solid" and seventy-pound weight loss, Peters decorates her text with punny jokes (Mrs. Weyaton and Mrs. Ima Gobbler are favorite characters) and cute drawings of rotund stick figures. *Diet and Health* quickly became and stayed a bestseller. By 1939, the book had sold two million copies and had been published in more than fifty-five editions.[31]

Peters dedicated *Diet and Health* to Herbert Hoover and invoked patriotic reasons for weight loss. Fat people hoarded calories desperately needed by American soldiers and European civilians, she explained; it was "unpatriotic to be fat." She also suggested creating a "Watch Your Weight Anti-Kaiser" program.[32] After serving with the American Red Cross in the Balkans, Peters grew more serious in her 1921 addendum describing her efforts to "raise funds for the starving children of Central Europe." She directly linked weight loss in the U.S. to desperate hunger abroad, asking dieters to think of hunger pangs as a "double joy, that of knowing we are saving worse pangs in some little children, and that of knowing that for every pang we feel we lose a pound."[33]

Books like these represent some of the earliest American diet plans, designed for everyday Americans and bundling ideas about health, diet, and food into larger political and ethical considerations. By eating less meat, wheat, and sugar, Americans would improve their health while serving their country and fulfilling a moral obligation to prevent starvation. These noble goals translated into specific recipes and methods of cooking, charging the ordinary routines of cooking and eating with greater purpose.

The work of Peters, Hoover, and Kellogg suggests the fluidity of diet and nutrition advice across disciplines and philosophies in the early twentieth century. Medical, political, and religiously motivated diet advice all drew from the knowledge created by these other fields: Kellogg used calories to advocate for purer spirits, Hoover claimed good health could be a side effect of the war effort, and Peters insisted a slim figure and patriotism went hand-in-hand. Early twentieth-century diet advice dealt in largely gender-neutral terms; however, in the years to come, diet advice split and different faddish or medical diets began to appeal to different types of health-conscious Americans.

Diet advice divided into two distinct and usually gendered camps in the twenty years from World War I through the Great Depression. In his history of fatness, Peter Stearns observes a similar shift toward feminine weight loss concerns, noting that prior entreaties targeted a more gender-neutral obesity characteristic of middle-class excess. After the Depression, discussions of overweight children also divided into underweight boys and overweight girls.[34] As Stearns puts it, "it was only in the 1920s that the more familiar gender contours surrounding dieting fully developed," directed at women's guilt rather than men's fears. Katharina Vester dates the distinction slightly earlier, suggesting that starting around the mid-nineteenth century, men—not women—were most concerned with weight loss and an ideal physique. A newly sedentary and industrialized society tested conventions of American masculinity; dieting demonstrated collective willpower and reinvigorated claims of biological superiority over women and nonwhite men.[35] Scared of sissification and unnerved by women's growing political power, American men began shoring up their manhood by growing beards, hunting big game, climbing mountains, and building muscle through systematic exercise regimens.

Men's exercise trends illustrate the beginning of this division in the 1910s and 20s. Called America's "most successful fitness guru," Bernarr "Body Love" Macfadden promised his raw foods and fitness plans would cure maladies from a cough to otherwise fatal cancers. Like Fletcher, Macfadden was an influential public figure, hobnobbing with Eleanor Roosevelt and, in an odd moment in American history, Benito Mussolini, who, after inviting

Macfadden to Rome, bragged about the fresh fruit—grapes, especially—in the Italian diet; Macfadden told Mussolini his soldiers ate too much.[36] Macfadden not only built an empire out of his *Physical Culture* magazine and spas but also created a legacy of male fitness gurus by mentoring Charles Atlas. Atlas, in turn, taught Jack LaLanne, best remembered today as the fitness leader so influential that Arnold Schwarzenegger called LaLanne "an apostle for fitness."

With masculine diet and exercise plans on one side, the new fad diets of the 1910s also split women's contributions to food reform into two camps: serious scientific nutrition in the emergent fields of domestic science and home economics on one side and fad dieting on the other. The term "fad diet" was popularized around World War I and these fad diets were dismissed as irrational, feminine, and ineffective, pooh-poohed by the government and domestic scientists alike. In contrast to Peters's more balanced diet, many of these new diets were food-specific. Bananas, grape juice, potatoes, or the pork-chop-and-pineapple plan were all in vogue.[37] Rice, macaroni, and milk were other "one-article" plans.[38]

Hollywood also helped. Silver screen glamor drove fad diets when Hollywood actresses promoted weight loss elixirs, reducing creams, and diet plans. Movie theater lobbies often featured penny scales, then an "icon of health and physical culture," beautifully constructed and adorned with images of glamorous starlets.[39] Celebrity endorsement reached its peak when Madame Sylvia of Hollywood, diet masseuse to the stars, was blacklisted for revealing celebrity secrets in her 1931 *Hollywood Undressed*, an exposé that doubled as a diet book and suggested helpful low-fat cooking techniques.[40] Dancer and starlet Wini Shaw pushed her "clock regime" of meal timing to lose twenty-five pounds in three months. Actress Jean Harlow promoted a diet of lamb chops, steak, Jell-O, and tomatoes to lose six pounds in four days.[41] Later, "Hollywood Special Formula Bread" ran cross-promotional advertising by featuring celebrities such as Elizabeth Taylor and Debbie Reynolds alongside the forty-six-calorie sliced bread. By 1935, Hollywood diets were so well entrenched that novelist Fannie Hurst criticized how the "standards of American Beauty are being set up and authorized by the bizarre little so-called civilization known as Hollywood." She listed the Hollywood "reduction fads" of the day: "skimmed-milk-and-baked-potato, the liquid bread, the thyrodic bath salt, the paraffin sweat, the holy rolling-machine," among others.[42]

Fad diets emphasized loveliness and beauty rather than simple weight loss; nutrition was rarely mentioned. A few diets promised "scientific eating" would "restore loveliness," but mostly a healthy body was a beautiful one. Earlier beauty food fads paved the way for one-article weight loss diets. As early as 1905, reports of "health and beauty dinners" served for high-society belles offered helpful tips. Olive oil and fruits lifted the spirit. Cooked grains produced a "peaches and cream complexion." The milk and vegetable diet brightened dull cuticles.[43] "Beautiful women are made of mayonnaise dressing," another authority claimed.[44] In the next few decades, these one-article diets became less cosmetic and more focused on weight loss. As they matured, fad diets presented good health as a dreamy mix of slenderness, beauty, and youth impossible to measure with a bathroom scale.

Pineapples and elixirs also sing of alchemy in a culture that so sternly insisted on science. Perhaps fad diets took off in the Progressive Era precisely because of domestic science, masculine scientific nutrition, and women's careful, no-nonsense conservation efforts during World War I. Matronly calorie-counters professionalized and rationalized a system which, at its heart, could be exciting, or at least rich material for the imagination. For young women, faddish pork-chop-and-pineapple diets may have been a method to rebel precisely because the persnickety diet authorities insisted on rationality. In fact, the authorities interpreted these one-food diets as a rebellion and publicly took offense to fad diets. The American Medical Association weighed in on "reduceomania" in a special 1926 session by "condemning the craze" and urging impressionable young women to instead follow a balanced diet. In 1935, Carl Malmberg published a scathing critique of reducing diets titled *Diet and Die*, a fitting title given his ominous warning that it is "better to be fat than dead."[45]

In the next few decades, serious diets continued to promote scientific nutrition. The USDA continued to release food guidelines, updating federal recommendations in 1933 to include a buying guide for different budgets.[46] Scientific, seemingly objective dieting may also have been a response to Nazi physical culture and fitness. The racist politics of the 1936 Berlin Olympics exposed Hitler's views on the physical superiority of the Aryan body and high-profile American Jewish and Catholic organizations publicly denounced Hitler's Aryans-only athletics.[47] The medical promotion of good nutrition perhaps appealed to Americans newly wary of the quest for physical perfection. Wartime food advice also simplified a sober, moderate approach to balanced nutrition. After President Roosevelt assembled the 1941 National Nutrition Conference for Defense, three new food guides advised Americans on good eating during wartime. In 1942, sugar became the first rationed consumer commodity, cutting prewar consumption in half by enforcing an average yearly ration of twenty-four pounds. Meat, lard, cheese, butter, and margarine soon followed, but surveys showed sugar outranking gasoline, steak, or butter as the most coveted good.[48] A comprehensive *National Food Guide* was reissued in 1946. The guide divided foods into the "basic seven" categories still familiar to Americans today: dairy, meat, bread, fat, and three categories of fruits and vegetables.[49] The foundation diet of basic food groups persisted as the core categories until the USDA replaced MyPyramid with MyPlate in 2011.

Medical research investigating the relationship of cholesterol to the "coronary plague" of heart disease also added seriousness to diet advice at this time.[50] The American Heart Association (AHA) reinvented itself in 1948 and began hosting high-profile celebrity fundraisers. Ancel Keys, the former chairman of the International Society of Cardiology and inventor of the K-ration, sparked the cholesterol wars in the 1950s. Nicknamed Mr. Cholesterol, Keys's advice to reduce cholesterol intake was heeded and margarine consumption trended skyward, later outselling butter in 1957.[51] When President Eisenhower suffered a heart attack in 1955, public concern was palpable and reporters widely publicized Eisenhower's low-cholesterol dry toast and Sanka diet.

Both the cholesterol wars and federal food policies were explicitly gendered male. From the outset in 1947, the AHA warned businessmen about the dangers of their high-stress, high-cholesterol lives. The AHA promoted its fundraising efforts with claims that heart disease first knocked down doctors, lawyers, and business executives. Men with heart disease were called "the successful failure. . . . But, like the busy bees, die off sooner than the rest of the hive." By 1955, as Keys wrote for *Time*, "The image of the tycoon who, at age 50, has attained money, success, a yacht, and a coronary thrombosis is almost part of American folklore."[52] Diet for heart disease was serious and lifesaving; diet for weight loss was superficial and self-indulgent.

Changes in food processing technology and the adoption of artificial sweeteners contributed to the split between serious, masculine health-promoting diets and self-indulgent feminine diets. Business interests gave women's diets a bad reputation when they peddled grape juice, gelatin, and cooking oil as diet aids. Cubbison Cracker Company published a party guide of "slenderizing menus" and Wesson's vegetable oil promised "glorious eating for weight watchers."[53] Artificial sweeteners, nonfat milk, and a slew of low-calorie cookies, candy, puddings, and ice cream mixes created a market of sweet-tooth dieters with seemingly little willpower. In 1956, one doctor explained that quack recipes will always be in vogue because "fat women so strongly desire to be fooled."[54] As historian Carolyn de la Peña observed, women began experimenting with noncaloric sweeteners in the late 1940s.[55] A 1954 article estimated that the nation's thirty million dieters could now "buy sweet things that contain no sugar, salty things minus the salt, starchy things low in calories."[56] Poppy Cannon, former *Ladies Home Journal* editor and widow of NAACP secretary Walter White, published *Unforbidden Sweets* in 1958. Designed for "weight-conscious gourmets," the cookbook contained recipes for "150 luscious low-calorie desserts" such as chartreuse of honeydew or orange chiffon pie. *Unforbidden Sweets* promised to "make your dessert-time a delight instead of a denial."[57]

Sweet foods and desserts, a category of "fattening" foods called "saccharine and farinaceous" in the eighteenth and nineteenth centuries and now categorized by their high carbohydrate content, most obviously differentiated feminine from masculine diets. Anthropologists have speculated as to the universality of the gendered associations between men, hunting, and meat versus women, gathering, and sugar. Scholar Amy Bentley argues the association runs deep between the "men/meat–female/ sugar dichotomy" in the contemporary American diet. Since the early nineteenth century, sugary, nutrient-poor foods have disproportionately constituted women's diets. To this day, women consume more sugars than men and studies show women more often crave sweets, ice cream, and cake and men prefer meats.[58]

Supposedly universal and natural, this dichotomy is political and bound up in the history of industrial capitalism. As Sidney Mintz has documented, sugar prices declined precipitously with the growth of Caribbean plantation slavery in the late eighteenth and early nineteenth centuries.[59] Slave labor created a cheap, accessible source of calories for the working classes in Britain. In general, control over and access to food (particularly applicable to the distinction between nutrient-poor sugar and nutrient-dense meat) helped maintain "class, caste, race and gender hierarchies," as Carole Couni-han explained in her study of food, gender, and power. She put it pithily, noting that "men eat first, best, and most."[60] Just around the same time sugar prices dropped, laymen like William Banting published high-protein, low-sugar diets for a wealthy male readership, formalizing the long-standing link between protein, class, and gender in one of the first diet manuals. Per-haps it wasn't by accident that cheap sugary foods first came to characterize women's diets in the nineteenth century and later differentiated diet books designed for women in the twentieth, upholding the gendered hierarchy of high-protein health advice against sweet, faddish diet books.

Sweetness became and is now still a defining characteristic of feminine diets, especially those promoted by food companies. Even as new diets challenged existing food industries, sugar refiners and producers of sweet foods retaliated with diets of their own. In 1933, a diet book subtitled *The Welch Way to Weight Control* discredited the argument that "grape juice is sweet and sweets are fattening" by explaining grape sugar is predigested and "is not stored by the body as fat." The company included recipes for "frozen dainties" and desserts such as grape whip, grape pudding, grape eggnog, and Welch's cornstarch pudding with marshmallow garnish to help diet-ers lose weight.[61] In 1942, the Sugar Research Foundation decried faddists and home economists whose diets posed "an active menace to the sugar industry," spreading unjust propaganda to "our feminine friends" in search of slimmer figures.[62] By the 1950s, sugar refiners ran advertising campaigns to promote sugar as a diet aid that supplied quick energy fast for a mere eighteen calories a teaspoon.[63] Unlike other reducing diets that demand "Spartan-like self-denial, and turn happy lives into martyred routines," the Domino Sugar Diet "contributes to the enjoyment of eating and makes your life more pleasant."[64] Associations of confectioners and bakeries also released advertising materials appealing to women by promoting candy and cakes as diet aids.

Before this schism between delight and denial was so firmly established, a woman like Lulu Hunt Peters could author a diet book and dedicate it (sin-cerely, and with permission) to a political figure as well regarded as Herbert Hoover. Afterward, it was rarer that a book could straddle the line between faddish and serious. Masculine medical diets were set explicitly against feminine fad diets like the housewife favorite 10-Day Miracle Diet. Severe, serious books like *The Low-Calory Cookbook* (1951) by Bernard Koten or

Norman Jolliffe's *Reduce and Stay Reduced* (1952) recommended punishing diets of very low-calorie meals, broken down by caloric content. The director of the New York City Bureau of Nutrition at the time, Norman Jolliffe includes an excruciatingly low 600-calorie-a-day menu of small quantities of skimmed milk, twenty-five-calorie-count bread, and four-ounce portions of flounder or lobster. Yet even a superficial reading reveals these serious books similarly emphasize how weight loss increases beauty. Jolliffe doesn't shy away from the aesthetic value of slenderness, claiming that weight loss will "simultaneously make you more attractive, feel better, and live longer." With a touch of defensiveness, Jolliffe writes in his introduction to *Reduce and Stay Reduced*, "It is a serious book on a deadly serious subject."[65]

The medical community did not question Jolliffe's disdain of "diets." One 1952 *American Journal of Public Health* review of Jolliffe's *Reduce and Stay Reduced* praised the book for opposing the "numerous quack cures, fad diets, and . . . various types of reducing aids." Unlike those "nostrums and reducing salons," *Reduce and Stay Reduced* contained accurate information, with scientific charts and tables, and could be recommended by all physicians.[66] Jolliffe and his contemporaries didn't just set themselves apart from feminine, faddish diets by tone or approach; they were actively unkind toward women. Jolliffe psychologized the overweight, blaming overbearing mothers who "nag, nag, nag" children to overeat. He hypothesized that "unmarried women" binge ate to dodge their "duties and responsibilities [as] wives and mothers" because few men would marry a fat woman.[67] This nastiness didn't go unnoticed and a few women book reviewers sideswiped his "pull no punches" technique or "unsmiling approach" that so spitefully blamed "Mme. Overweight."[68]

Food activism of the 1960s further widened the rift between so-called fad diets and serious food programs. The cholesterol wars were still being waged with the 1961 publication of the Framingham Heart Study findings that middle-aged men, in particular, were at risk for both elevated cholesterol and heart attack. Another, equally serious approach to food emerged at this time: the countercultural push for alternative food politics—vegetarianism, macrobiotics, back-to-the-land farming, consumer boycotts, interracial dining protests, antiwar fasts. The countercultural movement stressed food systems and diet as inherently political, inviting the individual into a larger ecological awareness about the production and distribution of food.

Cesar Chavez and other labor leaders brought farmworkers' rights into mainstream politics. The 1960 documentary *Harvest of Shame* publicized farmworker exploitation practices, and the subsequent United Farm Workers 1965–1970 grape boycott encouraged consumers to vote with their forks. Radical feminist vegetarian groups like the Bloodroot Collective insisted vegetarianism and natural foods supported their gynophilic and ecoconscious worldview.[69] Going back to the basics, however, often meant more work in the kitchen. Many feminists were suspicious of how home-baked bread or natural foods could both liberate women from domestic labor and fight against patriarchal repression.

This activism was a political world apart from 1960s weight loss diets. At the same time hippies were creating a "countercuisine," Jean Nidetch was growing Weight Watchers into an empire and artificially sweetened diet drinks ignited the new low-calorie market.[70] Some books straddled the political line. True to its title, Francis Lappé's bestselling *Diet for a Small Planet* was at once a political manifesto and a meal-by-meal menu. More than a million copies had been sold by the time the book went into its second edition in 1975. Lappé championed an environmental vegetarianism and railed against industrial agriculture while also offering a food plan. Even though the plan was not designed for weight loss, Lappé fixated on high-protein, low-calorie foods. Certainly many of Lappé's readers followed recipes for "Lentils, Monastery Style" or "Low-Calorie Cheese Spread" more for weight loss than political protest. In fact, when Lappé toured the talk show circuit, many of her hosts were quick to discuss the weight loss potential for this new diet.[71] Similarly, Susie Orbach's 1978 *Fat Is a Feminist Issue* promised to liberate women from the "merry-go-round" of "fat/thin" oppression by being an "anti-diet guide for permanent weight loss."[72]

Even as groups like the Bloodroot Collective championed antipatriarchal ways of eating, feminists believed that dieting was a tool of oppression that promoted unrealistic beauty ideals and shored up traditional gender roles. Though some scholars recast dieting as an assertion of agency, most feminists today agree that dieting is harmful to women and girls. Naomi Wolf has been one of the most outspoken feminists on the issue, claiming that "dieting is the most potent political sedative in women's history."[73] Others worry dieting internalizes self-surveillance in the Foucauldian sense, creating internal cycles of shame and disappointment. Structurally, many scholars agree that "diet discourses thus can be seen as serving the interests of a patriarchal social system, keeping women's attention directed towards the production of a docile body" even if the individual practices provide a temporary sense of control.[74] Yet others take a more complicated view toward dieting as a "multi-facetted practice that not only subjects the body to hegemonic cultural norms but simultaneously allows individuals to claim privileges."[75] Bodily control, however limited, is an act of assertion and self-control. Yet the fine line between dangerously disordered eating and dieting makes these earlier concerns particularly understandable. Anorexia often begins with a more benign dieting regimen and many feminists fear that, given the climate of impossibly thin beauty ideals, dieting can quickly devolve into an eating disorder.

Though often at odds with one another, the countercultural alternative food movements and medical diets saw faddish weight schemes as a common foe. Cabbage soup or banana diets were an easy target and many self-proclaimed experts ridiculed fads to legitimate their own plans as balanced and serious. In ways that mirror the masculine slant of the alternative food movement today, the language of dieting is easy to brush off as feminine and inconsequential while other types of food prescriptions—regulatory, health-seeking, medical, political—are legitimated by men. Even early manuals authored by women, such as Lulu Hunt Peters's 1918 *Diet and Health* and Mary Dickerson Donahey's 1923 *The Calorie Cook Book* are more often written into the history of domestic science than that of food history.

Around the 1990s, however, something changed again. Diets of the 1990s began taking a collective approach, looking holistically at the state of the nation and the health of its people from the perspective of the obesity epidemic. The American Heart Association declared a "war on fad diets" in 1997 because the diets failed to stem the tide of obesity. Diets of the 1990s look more like diets of the 1890s than diets in between for how they unite men and women, pledging the health of a nation against the strength of its people. Though fears of race suicide and feminization may have motivated the first wave of nineteenth-century masculine dieting, diets at the turn of the twenty-first century unite Americans in a gentler, more nostalgic utopian dream of racial and gender equality. *Fin de siècle* diets revered and perhaps fetishized the individual body—Bernarr Macfadden, Charles Atlas, the many fictional representations of Arrow Adonis—whereas contemporary diets reimagine the collective, looking back at an America that has been lost: a Paleolithic paradise, an American Eden, or precolonial, pre-industrial dreamlands.

Diets published since the 1990s have most often rejected an individualized etiology of obesity as a moral deficit for the belief that the obesity epidemic is a collective, community problem with common origins and common cures. All Americans—fat or thin—are implicated in the fight against obesity. Estimates about the public health burden of obesity costs have supported this logic. In 1992, a public health researcher analyzed 1986 data to warn of obesity's $39.3-billion bill levied on the American taxpayer. In 1995, that number nearly tripled to $99.2 billion when researchers combined the direct and indirect effects of the condition.[76] Obesity was also a global concern. After convening a special 1997 session on obesity, the World Health Organization (WHO) called obesity a "global epidemic" and "major global public health problem." The WHO also instituted a body mass index classification scheme labeling mildly overweight people as "pre-obese," signaling the universal susceptibility to the progression of overweight to obesity.[77]

The facts of the obesity epidemic are hotly contested. Categories of fat and thin, overweight and underweight necessarily depend on an idea of a normal weight, a fluid construct that varies widely across cultures, between individuals, and over time.[78] Obesity measurement methods are crude tools that rarely account for patterns of fat storage, muscle mass, age, race, and basic bodily variation between human beings. In 1998, the National Institute of Health (NIH) issued the first federal guidelines on obesity using body mass index (BMI) to categorize Americans according to weight while warning of heightened disease risk for those on the higher end of the scale.[79] BMI takes only height and weight into account, but with more sensitive criteria, standards change rapidly and push millions of Americans in and out of the overweight range. In 1998, the NIH lowered the BMI weight cutoff and suddenly twenty-nine million Americans became overweight without gaining a pound.[80]

Epidemiological studies of obesity likely account for this shift to the social and collective. Since 1970, calculated obesity rates have doubled from 15 to 30 percent of American adults.[81] In fact, this shift is best reflected in the term obesity "epidemic" itself, a term virtually unknown in discussions of overweight prior to 1990 and one that only lost its borrowed quotation marks around 1998. After 2000, the term was itself epidemic, growing from a paltry 650 hits in 1995–2000 newspapers to nearly 10,000 hits in news articles published between 2000 and 2005.[82]

By the time *The Surgeon General's Call to Action to Prevent and Decrease Overweight and Obesity* was issued in 2000, the language of epidemic was firmly embedded in public discussions of fat in the United States. Communication scholar Gordon Mitchell and epidemiologist Kathleen McTigue argued that the language of an "obesity epidemic" created "three interlocking rhetorical moves": to "impart urgency to the situation [by] tapping into society's collective memory of devastating infectious plagues," to reframe obesity from a cosmetic concern to a health issue, and to "facilitate understanding of excess body weight trends as a universalistic problem calling for a collective societal response."[83] Diet books quickly took up this collective societal response, potentially broadening the dieting population to people who newly fell into redefined categories of overweight and pre-obese and, drawing from the social contagion metaphor of epidemic, feared that they were at risk of becoming overweight without early intervention.

The rhetoric of epidemic also reunited the gendered camps of men's health advice and women's weight loss diets. Before the 1990s, male-authored diet books were typically more authoritative and standoffish. But with the onset of the epidemic, most diet books took on a more gender-neutral tone, signaled by an increasingly confessional and intimate masculine perspective, and universalizing language that appealed to all Americans—men or women, fat or thin. The concept of an obesity epidemic unified the various strains of food and health activism in American politics and culture and, in turn, created a unifying narrative of America's fall into obesity and disease. The "globesity" scare, or the fear that Americans have exported obesity abroad, adds a global lens to a discussion once limited to the Western world. What was once considered a disease of affluence is now more a scourge of the poor: obesity is strongly correlated with poverty in the United States and obesity rates are rising steadily in many non-Western countries. Many experts consider rising global obesity rates an aftershock of colonialism that indicates the corrosion of traditional values. These narratives are indebted to longer anthropological and literary discourses of primitivism and over-civilization, and diet books readily expose these debts to the rhetoric of Western decadence and decline.

Many scholars have questioned the uniformity of this narrative and have shown how expert advice to eat healthfully cannot be unaccompanied by grander schemes for the health of the body politic. As food studies scholar Katharina Vester has recently noted, "Cooking advice traditionally not only spread ideas about how to prepare dishes properly and healthfully (with reference to medical authority), but also circulated instructions on how to set tables, how to organize a household, how to treat servants, how to raise a family, and how to contribute to one's community and nation."[84] The growing field of academic food studies has taken this balance of power as a tenet of its academic inquiry. Since the early 2000s, food activism has rallied around a more diverse set of political concerns. Called the alternative food movement, members united a gourmet's approach to flavor, an environmentalist concern about sustainability, and more traditional left-leaning activism suspicious of industrial production, global capital, and federal regulation. Gourmets were recast as "foodies," a more politicized identity that appraised the deliciousness of food against the ethics and environmental sustainability of food origins.

Critics accuse the food movement of elitism, self-indulgence, and short-sightedness. They suggest alternative foodies are gourmets masquerading as activists, lefties that have left labor behind, and pleasure seekers that use politics to justify dessert. Yet a sensitive study of American food reform over the last hundred years reveals that today's critics are levying ungenerous accusations. Foodies unite factions of food reform in the United States that have always fought. Doctors accuse dieters of dangerous medical practices, activists attack gourmets for decadence, and everyone else blames lose-weight-fast fad dieters for promoting unhealthy body ideals, endangering young women, and for generally being misguided and irresponsible. The alternative food movement today unifies these disparate groups—doctors, politicians, environmentalists, and dieters—and the cabin fever infighting is simply more obvious now that they live under a single roof.

Perhaps this book should be read as a prelude to the present. Today, the authoritative meal-by-meal diet has matured into a more comprehensive system of food politics that uses weight loss as just one of its appeals for social or political change. Diets have always embedded weight loss in loftier narratives of positive change, but today's food movement upholds even grander goals—environmental, ethical, patriotic, national, moral—by relying on the higher sensibilities of the dieter. Instead of a lesson in calories and carbohydrates, this new food movement appeals to the softer stuff that makes us human beings: our experience of pleasure and our desire to do good. Real, natural, good, whole—these are the subjective categories Americans must define for themselves, an especially urgent task when "voting with your fork" raises the stake on every bite.

The food movement makes a study of diet books all the more urgent. Culture has never been contained between the covers of a book, but today's diet advice is subtle and shifty, embedded into everyday decisions of right and wrong. Contemporary diet books move beyond modern interpretations of age-old anxieties. They describe new and different ways of living, of thinking about the world and our place in it. Diet books are more screenplays than stories, narratives that millions of dieters live by, eat by, and believe in. And this book will show how diet books have served as a powerful and hugely accessible arena for the philosophical debate in America about who we are and how we should live.

1 ↣ PALEOLITHIC DIETS AND THE CAVEMAN UTOPIA

"LIFE WAS GOOD for our Paleolithic grandparents," recounts a 2001 diet book.[1] A 2013 diet laments that civilization has "transformed healthy and vital people free of chronic diseases into sick, fat, and unhappy people."[2] But, as one Paleo leader promised, "Eating Paleo can save the world."[3]

An estimated three million Americans currently follow some version of the Paleo diet and Paleo books are among the bestselling titles within an already blockbuster genre.[4] At its most basic, Paleo diets reject agricultural products such as cereals and sugars for foods that could have been hunted or gathered—mostly high-fat, high-fiber meats and plants. In practice, "going Paleo" means everything from the ordinary to the outlandish.[5] Some dieters avoid artificial light, eat raw beef, forsake shoes, let blood, intermittently fast, engage in polyamorous sexual relationships, and "adopt a primal attitude."[6] For others, the diet is just that—a diet of mainly meat and vegetables (occasionally fruits and legumes) adopted to lose weight or gain muscle. Most dieters practice Paleo to lose weight, but this "species-appropriate diet" allegedly cures over a hundred ailments ranging from Alzheimer's to anxiety, epilepsy to acne.[7]

Despite its popularity, the Paleolithic diet has received little scholarly attention. The diet is not merely a collection of weight loss manuals but a complex and controversial social movement, indebted to a long history of primitivist nutritional counsel, divided by bitter philosophical splits, and alternately mocked and praised by mainstream medicine. In fact, the whole weight loss narrative genre has much to offer utopia studies; in particular, the caveman diet offers an embodied utopian practice embedded within a powerful story of an original, lost Paleolithic paradise.

But the caveman diet is more than a myth of a lost golden age and more than a handbook for weight loss; the diets are at once a manual for the body, the self, and society. Known by many different names—the caveman, Stone Age, evolutionary, or hunter-gatherer diet—Paleolithic diets have been heralded as the best "way of life," a "revolution," and, most importantly, the "the first glimpse of a new and better world."[8] The Paleo diet differs from the perpetual processes of self-improvement characteristic of most self-help literature by linking corporeal and social transformation, enlisting the body to measure and materialize the processes of recouping the utopia within. These diets uphold social dreams with shared origins (in the cave), a collective problem (the obesity epidemic), and common ends (health for all). As the 2013 *The Paleo Manifesto* puts it, the diet aspires "to understand where we come from, to make the best of where we are, and to craft a better future."[9]

Such diets share the defining characteristic of many utopian visions— they are useful fictions. But this useful fiction is especially important to the body-utopia relationship because the caveman diet mixes myth and manual to create a new type of embodied utopia. Unlike medieval "body utopias" that relish excess, these caveman diets envision a new and different kind of body utopia characterized by calculated restraint and checked desire. By recalibrating the palate away from industrial foods, these foodways redefine pleasure as checked desire—not euphoric abandon. To borrow Ruth Levitas's language, the diet promises to "re-educate desire" by teaching the palate to resist the extreme flavors of modern foods and, instead, value and desire "natural" Paleo foods.[10]

This mix of myth and manual not only reveals how these dreams guide and exalt banal body practices, but also tells us about the worlds and bodies we dream of creating. In fact, the *place* of the promised paradise is actually the *body* of the dieter as the body brokers the bond between mythic history and utopian future. Most broadly, the story is told like this: since civilization (particularly agriculture) is such a recent invention on the timeline of human evolution, "our genes are still in the Stone Age" and we must "follow what our ancient ancestors ate" to recapture "our natural birthright of health."[11] In this narrative, the Paleo diet situates the individual body in the long, deep currents of human history, suggesting that the body is on loan from history and obliged to the future—and only one's own property for a short-lived half-blink of evolutionary time.

Nearly three decades ago, *The Paleolithic Prescription* opened with two questions: "Who are we? Where do we come from?"[12] In 2010, Robb Wolf asked in *The Paleo Solution*, "What were we like as hunter-gatherers, and what happened when we changed to agriculture?"[13] By 2013, the Ancestral Health Symposium convened six hundred caveman dieters to ponder the questions of "Where do we come from? Where are we going?" Paleo diets are part of a larger quest in American culture—the search for beginnings, the hunt for a homeland, the pursuit of a story that stakes its claim in where we come from to dream of where we should go.

THE CAVEMAN DIET SUBGENRE, OR, HOW BREAD IS THE STAFF OF DEATH

Western weight loss literature has a long tradition of venerating "primitive" diets and ways of life. In the eighteenth century, Jean-Jacques Rousseau proposed his "state of nature" theory of natural man. Extolling physical freedom and unfettered politics, Rousseau used primitive health to illustrate his theory of the natural goodness of mankind. Despite the hardships of tooth-and-claw life, Rousseau claimed that primitive man suffered from fewer sources of illness.[14] Since the nineteenth century, influential American diet reformers have conjectured about the diets of preagricultural peoples and recommended these "natural" foods to cure ailing moderns. In the 1890s, Dr. Emmet Densmore popularized a meat-heavy diet inspired by the "food of primal man," claiming that "bread is the staff of death" and "imbecility, decrepitude, and premature death go hand in hand with luxury and plenty."[15] To the dismay of vegetarian leaders, "primitive" diets were not restricted to Densmore's "anti-cerealism" or the low-carb cause.[16] Throughout his long life, Dr. John Harvey Kellogg (1852–1943) also speculated on "the ways and likings of our primitive ancestors of prehistoric times" to support his diet of grains and other farinaceous foods.[17]

Diet leaders have venerated the caveman—not simply the primitive— diet and ways of life since the 1920s. Between 1922 and 1924, French physiologist Charles Richet, the recipient of the 1913 Nobel Prize in Physiology and Medicine, promoted his raw meat tuberculosis cure, later called the "caveman" treatment in newspaper coverage.[18] Feeding tuberculosis patients pure raw meat juice produced encouraging results, ostensibly by reconstituting muscular tissues wasted by tuberculosis. In 1926, British surgeon Sir William Arbuthnot-Lane may have been the first to specifically recommend the "caveman's diet" as a nutritional role model. Speaking to packed auditoriums across the United States, Arbuthnot-Lane insisted that all diseases were the "terrible price for civilization" since poor health directly resulted from civilized nutrition.[19]

Like Kellogg and Densmore, Richet and Arbuthnot-Lane called civilization the cause of disease and nature the cure. Unlike Kellogg and his contemporaries, however, early twentieth-century proponents of the "cavemen cure" used a modified vision of Darwinian thought and evolutionary history to speculate on humankind's collective origins. Medical leaders often blurred these intellectual boundaries by alternately praising "pagan races" and man's Paleolithic ancestors for their nutritional superiority.[20] Until the 1970s the term "caveman" was often shorthand for a meaty or low-carbohydrate diet that could refer to either contemporary "primitive" or Paleolithic peoples. In 1975, the Seattle gastroenterologist Walter Voegtlin self-published *The Stone Age Diet*, the first full-length caveman diet, and solidified the school of thought into a distinct subgenre of diet literature (Figure 1.1). A little-known treatise on the health dangers of civilization, *The Stone Age Diet* narrates the now-familiar story of Paleolithic man straying from "his narrow dietetic path," acquiring the "doubtful assets of civilization," and falling victim to heart disease, gallstones, and obesity. Voegtlin recommended a "meat-fat" Stone Age diet of unlimited fish, meat, cheese, and eggs. He forbade starches, sweets, and vegetables like cabbage, cauliflower, radishes, and onions. Dieters could only drink "coffee, tea, postum, sour cream (NO

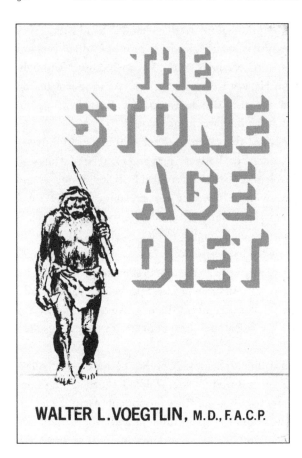

FIGURE 1.1. Walter Voegtlin's self-published *The Stone Age Diet* is considered the first full-length Paleo diet book.

MILK), buttermilk, whiskey and water."[21] Only five of the 277 pages of *The Stone Age Diet* describe the actual diet; the rest is a long manifesto about the dangers of civilization and the true way to primitive health.

There is a noticeable historical gap in caveman-themed diet advice between the Great Depression and the late 1960s. The diet itself might explain the interlude: two landmark low-carbohydrate plans bookend the period, coinciding with the first flash of 1920s interest in caveman diets and the later program sparked in the 1970s and expanded in the early 2000s. Arctic explorer Vilhjalmur Stefansson's 1913 *My Life with the Eskimo* and the 1921 *The Friendly Arctic* drew from his experience with the Inuit to popularize an all-animal diet to a broad American public. As the 1919–1922 president of the Explorer's Club, Stefansson also lectured across the United States promoting his blubber and organ meat diet for optimal health. After the 1920s, calorie-counting and more grain-based approaches elbowed out the low-carbohydrate diet until 1972, when Robert Atkins published his landmark *Dr. Atkins' Diet Revolution: The High Calorie Way to Stay Thin Forever*.[22] The 1972 book sold well but, more importantly, paved the way for the 1992 *Dr. Atkins' New Diet Revolution*, a book that spent five years on *The New York Times* bestseller list and is "among the top fifty bestselling books in history."[23] Like Atkins, Voegtlin pioneered a low-carbohydrate diet but distinguished his approach by "consider[ing] the matter of diet philosophically." Noting the high stakes, Voegtlin recruits dieters and warns the irresolute that they "must be imbued with the crusader's zeal, the single-mindedness of a martyr and a 'do or die' resolve."[24]

Changing representations of the Stone Age and cavemen might also account for the lull. The 1925 Scopes Monkey Trial politicized evolutionary theory and upset a fragile assimilationist peace, pitting ideas of modern science against fundamental Christian beliefs about mankind's origins. Such a fiercely partisan theological contest may have dissuaded Americans from embracing a caveman-inspired diet. News coverage of the trial depicted unflattering portraits of hirsute, comical brutes, and archaeological discoveries of Neanderthal remains in Africa reinforced racist beliefs about inferiority. *The Lost World*, a popular 1925 film, dramatized white men defeating vicious "ape-men."[25] Though the antimodern veneration of the primitive persisted, especially after the bloody combat of the first modern war degraded claims of an enlightened civilization, the caveman himself became a less-than-attractive model for a diet.[26]

Fluctuations in ideal body size and shape can also explain the fickleness in diet popularity more broadly. Most social historians of dieting agree that "middle-class America began its ongoing battle against body fat" at the turn of the twentieth century, between 1890 and 1910.[27] The turn-of-the-century "slimming craze" is most memorable in the slim, long-legged, flat-chested, athletic body ideal of the 1920s "flapper," a marked contrast to the busty, wasp-waisted Victorian.[28] Though historians of the period often focus on women's quest for new body ideals, both presidents of the period were scrutinized for their bodies. As Michael Kimmel observes, Theodore Roosevelt's "triumph over his own youthful frailty and his transformation into a robust vigorous man served as a template for a revitalized American social character."[29] The strenuous life president was replaced in office by William Howard Taft, a man ridiculed for his corpulence and "one of the first public figures in U.S. history to be defined popularly in terms of his pathologic obesity."[30] Like many young women of the period, Taft dieted throughout the 1910s and 20s.

From this initial interest in dieting, the mid-1930s to the 1960s interlude in caveman or low-carbohydrate diets reflects the events that dampened the appeal of dieting and weight loss more broadly. World War II food rationing and shortages temporarily interrupted the wave of fad diets. Americans weary of the savagery of war might have also preferred to celebrate modernity—civilized, clean, processed foods—rather than dwell on mankind's baser appetites. Organized, efficient TV dinners can be cast as the clean counterpoint to the bloody Paleo-style diet of meat and minimally processed fruits and vegetables. The postwar period also "revived the hourglass figure," with an idealization of more maternal, busty proportions.[31] Many favored the Marilyn Monroe look until the late 1960s and early 70s, when "Twiggy and Jean Shrimpton began to set a new norm for ultra-slenderness."[32] Most historians agree that the vicissitudes of American body ideals reflect larger concerns about the American character or body politic—usually concerns of "health" that include more abstract principles of strength, temperance, and nature.

More broadly, both forms of diet advice—either explicitly Paleolithic or largely primitive—belong to a broader strain of antimodernism in American instructive literature. Especially relevant is what R.W.B. Lewis identifies as the paradox that the "more intense the belief in progress towards perfection, the more it stimulated a belief in present primal perfection."[33] As a plan for a perfect future, Paleo diets reminisce on an unspoiled past to create a unifying concept of social, medical, and bodily reform. Paleo diets have long been bound into larger political and social visions and the reverence for the caveman speaks to a broad-spectrum critique of progress and civilization. In his time, Kellogg's anti-masturbation crusades and pantheistic sunflower worship won him greater fame than his cereals. In 1975, Voegtlin's dietary advice—eat double portions of meat, with lots of mayonnaise and buttermilk—was largely secondary to what was, at its core, a political manifesto about eugenics and race supremacy.

Paleo leaders today have tried to salvage the wheat of nutritional advice from the chaff of Voegtlin's unpalatable politics, but, like many diet books, *The Stone Age Diet* is more a political manifesto than a weight loss manual. Voegtlin was gripped by the fear that "our population is exploding everywhere faster and faster." He predicted a global population of twenty-five billion and, to combat famine and Malthusian catastrophe, Voegtlin recommended the "euthanasia of imperfect newborns" and birth control to limit "reproduction to superior types of individuals." In a creative take on Malthus, he uses the same logic to recommend eating tigers, dolphins, and other carnivores.[34] Man must also make a tough choice to "either eliminate them or eat them," referring to the large vegetarian animals that compete indirectly with man like elephants, giraffes, horses, and hippopotamuses. The "population explosion *is* here at hand," Voegtlin claims, and superior humans cannot allow weaklings or fish-eating mammals to consume precious resources. "Will [dolphins] be eliminated, or will man?" Voegtlin asks his readers, gesturing toward an apocalypse in which dolphins, fat on fish, overrun the world with their well-fed populations.[35]

Disagreeable or eccentric views like these dominated discussions of the "caveman diet" until a January 1985 *New England Journal of Medicine* article on Paleolithic nutrition by S. Boyd Eaton and Melvin Konner, both distinguished medical doctors with anthropological training, advanced the "evolutionary discordance hypothesis."[36] The discordance or "mismatch" hypothesis theorizes that the clash between "ancient body and modern world" produces obesity, diabetes, and the other "diseases of civilization" or, as they are sometimes called, diseases of affluence, longevity, environment, or lifestyle.[37] Broadly, Eaton and Konner argue that since "the human genetic constitution has changed relatively little since the appearance of truly modern human beings, *Homo sapiens sapiens*," preagricultural diets are the "nutrition for which human beings are in essence genetically programmed."[38]

More specifically, Eaton and Konner advance two important and controversial claims that still provide the theoretical backbone of the Paleo movement today. First, Eaton and Konner argue divisively that the human body has remained essentially unchanged since the Paleolithic era.[39] Second, they cite evidence that preagricultural people were, on average, "six inches taller than their descendants who lived after the development of farming" to argue that the "invention of agriculture" led to poor health.[40] Effectively, Eaton and Konner refute the "nasty, brutish and short" critics who cited brief Paleolithic life expectancy (roughly estimated from twenty to forty years) to claim that Paleolithic people died before they could contract the diseases of civilization, usually chronic degenerative conditions accompanying old age or senescence.[41]

Eaton and Konner's views generated great controversy in the late 1980s and are still fiercely debated in medical, anthropological, and evolutionary scholarship and the popular press. Yet a holistic plan of Paleolithic nutrition did not coalesce until 2002 when Dr. Loren Cordain published *The Paleo Diet: Lose Weight and Get Healthy by Eating the Foods You Were Designed to Eat*, now considered the cornerstone of the Paleo movement. Eaton and Konner's research directly inspired Cordain, creating what the author calls "the defining moment in my career, which set me off on a 30-year quest" and led to "a worldwide concept now known as 'The Paleo Diet.'"[42] Cordain's 2002 book has been translated into more than twenty languages and, as he asserts, "the term Paleo has become a household word since the publication of my first book."[43] Mark Sisson created his Paleo blog in 2006 with the "mission is to change the lives of ten million people"; the site now receives an estimated 2.5 *million* unique visitors in web traffic every month.[44] By 2009, the Ancestral Health Society (AHS) officially organized to offer a "new direction in physiology that respects our heritage as human beings."[45] Google announced that Paleo was the most searched for diet in 2013, even as *U.S. News & World Report* ranked the controversial diet last on its list of "Best Diets Overall."[46]

Given the recent explosion in interest, the bibliography leans heavily toward contemporary books. My research draws from the close reading of thirty-five primary books roughly categorized as Paleo diets from 1975 to 2017, with particular attention to the three "fathers" of the Paleo movement: Walter Voegtlin, S. Boyd Eaton, and Loren Cordain. This literary analysis is supplemented with internet resources and a dozen interviews with dieters, diet authors, and other self-identified ancestral health adherents.

SCHOLARSHIP ON THE BODY, GENDER, AND UTOPIA

Utopianist scholarship provides valuable insight into the meaning and practice of caveman diets. Lyman Tower Sargent has noted that "utopia is a tragic vision of a life of hope."[47] Powerfully, he shows how mythic utopias create an "inevitable dialectic of hope, failure or at least partial failure, despondency and the rejection of hope, followed in time by the renewal of hope."[48] We can "hope, fail, and hope again," living out what Sargent calls "the dialectic [that] is part of our humanity."[49] Without hope and a vision of original goodness, "we are left, not with a mature tragic spirit, but merely with a sterile awareness of evil uninvigorated by a sense of loss," R.W.B. Lewis noted.[50] And, indeed, the caveman diet deeply speaks to the literature and practice of this dialectic: of hope and failure, of the quest for ideal health and the inevitability of our mortality, of the desire to escape time and our certain incorporation into its currents.

By freeing the caveman within and recapturing "our natural birthright of health," paleo dieters plot themselves into an old history that starts fresh, beginning with the very beginning of mankind. Friedrich Nietzsche described something like this universal human search for a "lost paradise . . . that has nothing yet of the past to disown" to escape the "great and continually increasing weight of the past."[51] He urged Germans to practice forgetting the past. Early on, American studies scholars identified this as the pervasive myth of the "American Adam." R.W.B. Lewis elaborates that the myth "described the world as starting up again under fresh initiative in a divinely granted second chance for the human race, after the first chance had been so disastrously fumbled in the darkening Old World." The myth "saw life and history as just beginning," pioneered by the "hero of the new adventure: an individual emancipated from history" like Adam before the Fall.[52] F. O. Matthiessen called it the "frequent American need to begin all over again from scratch."[53] For many Americans, this need has been met by the vision of the Western frontier, a place Frederick Jackson Turner famously claimed was essential to the making of American democracy and character. Paleo diets replay the cave as the frontier, cheerfully insisting that dieters can begin from the beginning of recorded time and remake their bodies, lives, and worlds anew.

The Paleo myth is acted out on the stage of the dieting body. Returning to this mythic caveman past means releasing a health "sealed into our genes millions of years ago" and "embedded" in our modern bodies.[54] Usually utopian communities are built in the material world—communes like Oneida or Brook Farm come to mind—but as scholar Louis Marin reasons referring to "utopic Rabelaisian bodies," the "body is also a space and an architectural construction of sites and places."[55] This place-as-body recognizes what Ruth Levitas calls the "deliberate ambiguity" of the translation of Thomas More's *Utopia* as *outopia*—"no place"—or *eutopia*—"good place."[56] The place promised by the caveman utopia is less a built environment or social space than it is a state of body—the "good no place" of the living, unfinished site of the perfectible body. The diet book uses both the material of the body-as-space and the measure of the body-in-time to create a lived vision of embodied utopia. The body-in-time uses the instrument of the body to measure time much like Bakhtin suggests Rabelais used the body as a "concrete measuring rod for the world" which swirls around it.[57] The "present" material of the caveman dieter's body brokers between past and future in the metaphor of body reduction—or time measured by pounds lost.

Scholars have noted that "the concept of 'embodied utopia' may appear to be a contradiction in terms—with the body signifying unpredictability, concreteness and change, and utopia characterized by predictability, abstraction and permanence."[58] However, these researchers are not suggesting the incompatibility of concrete body and abstract utopia but indicating how useful a medium the body is for the concrete rendering of utopia—a living measure by which utopian dreams are literalized. This chapter approaches the same utopia-body relationship from the other direction—from the body to the world it promises to produce. Diets demonstrate how valuable the body is to the production of utopia because, as Eaton and colleagues put it, "the past resides within us."[59] The body of the caveman dieter is used as a tangible, concrete key to unlock interior utopias.

The Paleo diet also complicates the connections between gender and dieting. Ever since Susan Orbach declared that "fat is a feminist issue" in the late 1970s, scholars such as Susan Bordo and Kathleen LeBesco have revealed how the "commodification of thinness" reinforces existing hierarchies and hurts women in the impossible quest for the body ideal.[60] Unlike most diets, Paleo narratives often imagine the body as distinctively male and virile, using terms like "warrior" or "protector" to describe the strong, heroic body. Men may be the presumed audience for most Paleo books but, perhaps unsurprisingly for a diet, one Ancestral Health Society survey found that more women than men practice Paleo.[61] The Paleo veneration of the young, fit, white male body legitimates the diet: instead of just another faddish pursuit of a bikini body, the Paleo diet is cast as a lifestyle or fitness plan. Scholars have observed that men reject feminine food, such as, for example, when "middle class masculinity came under fire for being too soft and sedentary" in the early twentieth century. In response, American "authors borrowed from nostalgic imagery of the ways of life of the cowboy and the soldier to embrace campfire cooking."[62] Paleo leader Nell Stephenson even invented the word "Paleoista" to avoid the "'Cavie' approach," a term for "feminine, fit, and fantastic" women who find Paleo a "little too primal for my taste."[63]

Paleo leaders have also fought for the recognition of women's appetites, particularly for meat and other hearty "masculine" foods that are mainstays of Paleo diets.[64] Women's appetites have long been identified as both metaphor and method for patriarchal control; Susan Bordo observes that "the representation of unrestrained appetite" is "inappropriate for women," who are more often depicted nibbling on dainty, sweet little tidbits.[65] Even as Paleo women still restrict their diet to "acceptable" or "Paleo" foods, they assert their full appetites. As one Paleo enthusiast insisted, "I will continue to eat my steak, or roast, and I will enjoy it, very much. . . . I don't consider eating meat to be a gender specific thing, though. I consider it to be a human thing."[66]

Although feminist scholarship may challenge their political claims, Paleo leaders, in unlikely alliance, have identified with antidiet activism. Like these activists, Paleo women reject equations of beauty with thinness; one nutritionist even promised that Paleo helps women "form a healthy relationship with food" and "break the diet-sabotage cycle."[67] They insist that Paleo "is not a diet, but a lifestyle choice" or "that this was not a 'diet' but rather a complete lifestyle change."[68] Unlike antidiet and size-acceptance feminists, Paleo women simply cut a different ideal body shape from the same cloth. In keeping with the general shift toward athleticism since the 1980s, Paleo women swap the slender ideal for the strong one, rather than broadening feminine beauty ideals to a diversity of shapes, abilities, and sizes.[69] Skinny is not enough for the *Cavewomen Don't Get Fat* diet that describes a "skinny-fat" woman "who might look good in clothes" but, "in spite of her thin physique, she may still be jiggly and even have cellulite."[70] As another Paleo diet book explained, the cavewoman "might look like a supermodel, but not a skinny, starved waif—more Cindy Crawford than Kate Moss."[71]

However superficial the body ideals, a close analysis of the Paleo diet does reveal a vision of naturally more equitable cavepeople gender relations. This paradise overturns ideas of a "caveman masculinity," a concept used to naturalize gender differences and essentialize masculine domination. Paleo practice and diet books contradict familiar representations of the caveman as a belligerent thug who excuses his worst behavior with some weak pretext of biological compulsion, as all too commonly seen in titles such as 2009's *Why Women Love Cavemen—A Man's Guide to Tame the Bitch*. The self-published book teaches men how to "unleash your relentless power over her," even to "pull her hair and force her."[72] Not all caveman-themed self-help books are so ugly. David Clarke's 2007 Christian marriage advice book, *Cinderella Meets the Caveman*, describes primitive masculinity as both urge-driven ("Your Caveman loves food") and also gentle and respectful toward women ("You Are the Man. . . . Caveman, it's your job to lead her in every area of your relationship"). Clarke integrates evolutionary and Christian essentialist concepts by reminding his readers of Ephesians 5:22–24: "Wives, be subject to your own husbands, as to the Lord."[73]

Images of "club-wielding, wife-beating brutes" have led Martha McCaughey and other scholars to categorize the "caveman mystique" as a "popular embodied ethos of manhood" that naturalizes a loutish, sexually aggressive masculinity.[74] In John Pettegrew's terms, this type of "de-evolutionary masculinity" naturalizes antisocial behaviors, particularly those of male sexual violence.[75] Citing Pierre Bourdieu, Pettegrew shows how evolutionary psychology and, in turn, a caveman masculinity, participate in the "*relative dehistoricization* and *eternalization* of the structure of sexual division." For Bourdieu, the privileging of male biology "*legitimates a relationship of domination by embedding it in a biological nature that is itself a naturalized social construction.*"[76]

However, many Paleo books such as Eaton et al.'s *The Paleolithic Prescription* explicitly counter the "sexist images about our 'caveman' past: Alley-Oops [who] drags Betty-Boop (or whomever) along by the hair," by arguing for a "more balanced theory" of cavepeople gender relations.[77] More like the paradisiacal feminist landscape of Charlotte Perkins Gilman's *Herland* than Tarzan's jungle, Eaton and colleagues' vision of Paleolithic times upholds the "complementary roles, not dominance" of "Woman the Gatherer" and "Man the Hunter." "Women can and should have it all," the authors claim. "They were meant to, and did so for most of the time people have been on earth."[78]

Surprisingly, the Paleo diet also advances a vision of racial parity. On the face of it, the language of shared ancestry and biological uniformity could intimate a racist vision of the Übermensch. However, the vast scale of the Paleo narrative suggests otherwise. From the zoomed-out perspective of the grand narrative of human evolution, the individual differences of race, color, and national origin blur and become trivial. For example, while nodding to food allergies and genetic difference, Cordain still insists "we're all the same. We've all got the same basic human genome, shaped by more than

2 million years of evolution."[79] "Hunter gatherers are us," one diet explains, and "this book is a story about us. You know, *H. Sapiens*."[80] Another author reasons that, since tigers don't eat grass and rabbits don't eat meat, dieters must identify first as people, asking themselves, "Is this food natural for *human beings?*"[81] Another vivid passage from *Paleo Dog* argues that "humans show very little difference in the basic structure and function of the digestive system among racial groups."[82] When *Homo sapiens* are compared to rabbits and dogs, people look more similar than different—and this large-scale categorization of humans as hairless bipedal mammals, together with the spirit of the Paleo vision, contributes to a vision of equality and human unity.

Paleo diet books also bridge between two fields of utopian cultural productions: utopian literature and utopian practice. As a text—and a story with beginning, middle, and end—the diet book narrates what Darko Suvin calls an "alternative historical hypothesis" of human origins.[83] Unlike some utopias, the caveman diet doesn't merely offer "an explanation of how the better society came into being" but actually indicates "how that society was or could be achieved."[84] The practices of eating, sleeping, and exercising double as a plan to achieve the Paleolithic society—or at least its health, friendship, and leisure—and many dieters evaluate and live their lives by this mythic metric.

Yet these two fields—the practices prescribed by the diet and the story it narrates—are not simply two discrete chunks, easily severable and analyzable on their own terms. Rather, they reside in productive tension with one another: dieters decide how to practice Paleo by evaluating their daily habits according to the diet narrative and, in turn, they evaluate the narrative in light of their daily diet practice. Considering that "mammoths, aurochs, and mastodons are long since extinct," Eaton's team asks, "is it possible to eat as our ancestors did 25,000 years ago?"[85] Like most diet leaders, Eaton and his coauthors hedge their answer, using the concept of "equivalence" to substitute mastodons for other land mammals like cows, for instance, or pigs.

Most dieters vacillate less, sticking strictly to their own story of a lost Paleolithic past as they actively interpret and engage with the stories, often in the many interactive forms of self-evaluation that dot the diet book—questionnaires, body mass index (BMI) charts, and food diaries. For example, bitter arguments about dairy and legumes characterize two big splits in the Paleo community; purists insists that "docile, milkable cows" are a modern invention but one dieter told me, in a hushed tone, that since she loves

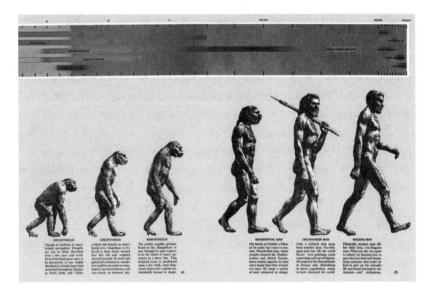

FIGURE 1.2. The iconic *March of Progress* by Rudolph Zallinger originally appeared in Time-Life's 1965 book *Early Man* and depicted a linear progression from apelike ancestors to modern man. Long criticized for wrongly portraying evolution as a parade toward a perfect state, the *March of Progress* is an iconic representation of evolution and often parodied in popular culture.

dairy, her vision of perfect health lay sometime in human history between the domestication of cattle and the invention of agriculture.[86] Another dieter similarly reinterpreted the Paleo vision because, contrary to Cordain's prohibition, she insisted, "I don't care if they [peanuts] are technically legumes, to me they are nuts because our ancestors could just dig them up, right?"[87] For most dieters, the Paleo narrative is more than a utopian blueprint or prospectus but rather a living document that is consulted, read, reread, interpreted, and reinterpreted in their daily lives.

All these concrete, real-life practices are driven by a literary origin story that narrates our collective origins, laments our decline, and promises an ideal world. Visually, this ascent-descent-promise-of-utopia story is represented in the familiar "March of Progress" scientific illustration that condenses twenty-five million years of evolution into a single image: from left to right, from lowly *Pliopithecus* and *Paranthropus*, slowly rising to Cro-Magnon Man to, finally, crescendo in upright, muscular *Homo sapiens sapiens* or Modern Man (Figure 1.2).

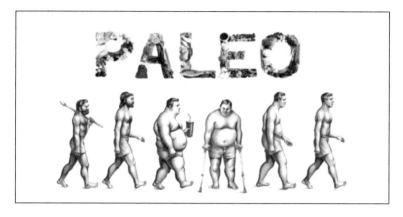

FIGURE 1.3. Paleo diets commonly riff on the iconic *March of Progress* by providing a sequel to the original 1965 scientific drawing. Mankind may have descended into obesity and disease but, as this illustration makes clear, the Paleo diet can recuperate older ways of health and reenlist mankind into the continual march toward a better future.

The Paleo diet illustrations riff on the March of Progress to show *descent* from our ancient ancestors—the pot-bellied, feminized contemporary man descending from a virile ancestor. Some illustrations leave the future unwritten, showing only present decay with a slovenly, overweight man at the rightmost final position. More often, however, the illustration shows how Paleo dieting will restore mankind's original strength. Figure 1.3, for example, symbolizes rock-bottom in the obese middle figure (the fourth in the left-to-right series), hobbled on crutches. The fourth figure is the only one to face the viewer head-on. He averts his gaze, downcast, even as his body confronts the viewer as if to display the full failure of his crippled, fat body. To his left, however, the succeeding stages of Paleo diet success are strong and purposeful, marching straight into the hope awaiting mankind at the right-hand margins of the future.

These images suggest what is much more explicit in the text—that the diet is a story about humanity, about evolution, about civilization and disease. The body of the individual dieter is situated in a long, deep history of mankind. The dieter is biologically indebted to the Paleolithic Era and, in turn, the coming generations will be indebted to him. Everyday body practices of the individual—eating, sleeping, walking—are elevated to symbols of mankind's ascent or descent, failure or triumph, in the grand narrative of progress. In this mix of myth and manual—or literature and practice—the diet book imbues the banal processes of embodiment with the utopic and recognizes what Ruth Levitas sees as a "praxis-oriented" form of concrete utopia which "refers forward to the emergent future."[88] The messy realities of the body-in-flux—the eating, slenderizing, strengthening body—gestures towards the "unfinishedness of the material world," which as Levitas frames it, "does not consist only of what is, but includes what is becoming or might become."[89]

FROM BODY TO BODY POLITIC, SELF TO SOCIETY

This collective vision of the body challenges what Victoria Pitts and other scholars have noted as "the modern Western body understood not as a collective product of inscription, but as a personal projection of the self."[90] Similarly, Anthony Giddens has marked the shift away from the modern "given," predetermined body to the postmodern body, available to be "'worked upon' by the influences of high modernity" and enlisted into the "reflexive project of the self."[91] Undoubtedly, the ideal Paleo body is part of this project of the self—it is sun-browned, virile, athletic, energetic, loving, clear-headed, with a fine-tuned palate and a keen set of instincts. However, the Paleolithic diets argue this better body makes the better world, as the improving self creates an improved society, with personal and social transformations that go hand-in-hand.

The link between body and world is often more fanciful than factual, but Paleo leaders insist that the health of one body inspires and contributes to social health. Or, as one Paleo webpage quoted, "You make the world a better place by making yourself a better person."[92] The Paleo Foundation claims: "We envision a healthier world. . . . We firmly believe that the Paleo Movement holds the key to changing the world."[93] Specifically, the Paleo Foundation describes the "key" as "supporting better animal husbandry practices," incentivizing "sustainable farming," and offering "continuous education."[94] Others are political: one Paleo business insisted their vision "incorporates a conscious effort to improve our social, economic and environmental wellbeing" by raising "awareness about the health benefits of the Paleo Diet while increasing access to locally produced wild and grassfed food."[95] Other Paleo practices incorporate political activism—primarily, the vituperative campaigns to legalize raw or nonpasteurized milk and abolish U.S. farm subsidies of grains.[96]

Many dieters also refer to environmental or social imperatives, explaining that the diet fulfills a "moral obligation" to the planet and fellow human beings.[97] One diet author dedicated her book to "my children . . . their unborn children, and those generations to come."[98] One dieter told me she "went Paleo" because "we are in a crisis point with the planet, with environmental sustainability," equating, as *Primal Cuisine* does, "sustainable body, sustainable earth."[99] More broadly, *Paleo Desserts* promises natural food that "allows you to live in harmony with planet Earth" while enjoying desserts like flax muffins and poppy-seed hot fudge sundae cake.[100] Though most experts agree that "the environmental impacts of meat" degrade water and soil, Paleo dieters refute these claims by blaming grain-fed livestock and monocultural agricultural methods—not "natural" Paleo free-roaming foraging animals and wild plants.[101]

However shaky these claims, leaders insist that Paleo is not merely an individual plan for self-improvement but a collective solution to a species-wide health crisis, broadly defined. This logic suggests what James Kopp has called a "medical utopia," visions that intertwine political thought with public health, demonstrating how the improvement of an individual's health creates a better society.[102] Health, in this sense, encompasses the health of the body and the body politic, most often emphasizing the leisure, kinship, decommodified "natural" economies, and equitable gender relations of the revitalized Paleo society.

MYTHS OF HUMAN ORIGINS AND THE PALEOLITHIC PARADISE

If the body harbors this Paleolithic heritage of health within it, what exactly does the alternative caveman society look like? And where is the Paleolithic period situated on this mythic chronology of human evolution? Most Paleo leaders ostensibly adhere to the scientific timeline of the roughly 30,000-year period from when humans evolved in 40,000 BC to the invention of agriculture in 10,000 BC.[103] Some Paleo dieters creatively interpret this timeline to accommodate creationist theories of human genesis by arguing that Adam and Eve either predate *or* descend from cavemen. One article reconciled creationism and evolution with the following: "Adam and Eve: The Father and Mother of the Paleo Diet," a view echoed in the 2011 *Original Thin* and even Eaton *et al.*'s first book.[104] One diet takes a particularly creative approach to the imaginary chronology of human development: the author situates ancient Paleo before "Biblical Times" and "American Indians," "Yoga," any "Large city or town," the "Growing of Crops," and even "Polynesians," among others.[105]

Despite variation in *when* humans lived as healthy cavemen, *what* this paradise looked like is largely uniform. In most caveman diets, "our ancestral homeland" is a prehistoric dreamland characterized by health, community, friendship, and a natural division of leisurely labor. Some diets advance more esoteric visions of primitive justice and denunciations of slavery or, in the tradition of the jeremiad, see our fallen obese state as punishment for prior misdeeds. Most, however, envision our caveman past as Eaton and colleagues do in their 1988 *Paleolithic Prescription*, which encourages the dieter to "suppose for a moment that you and your family" lived long ago, "back through unimaginable lengths of time . . . not just to Noah and Adam but to a place and time 40,000 years ago."[106] This time travel returns dieters to a pre-Edenic life of "closeness and interdependence" abounding with "talking, arguing, laughing, and playing."[107] They describe a day full of sweet honey, beautiful women, and abundant feasts; when the sun sets, "at last only the sound of a healer playing a stringed instrument and singing plaintive songs gives voice to the deep quiet of the night."[108]

Imagining ourselves back in our hunter-gatherer shoes (or bare feet), Sisson asks, "How did they fill a typical day?" Sisson describes "a life of physical challenge but ample leisure . . . living by the natural ebb and flow of lightness and darkness, season to season." In their "vast amounts of leisure time," "children would play. Babies and toddlers would nurse." At night, Sisson explains, "They would sing. Many would dance. Other nights might bring well-known and welcome stories around the intimacy of a fire circle. Beyond the circle there would be little to watch on most nights but the stars and the dim silhouette of a darkening landscape, the nearby sound of the wind in the grasses and, in the distance, calls of animals."[109]

Even hunting—a very unusual utopian feature—is tinted with a rosy glow.[110] After instructing readers to "imagine yourself travelling back in time—far back," *Paleo Diet—Good or Bad?* describes a bison hunt in loving detail. Unlike the "fowls that fly ready-roasted" in the Land of Cockaygne, the *Paleo Diet—Good or Bad?* recounts how, after "everyone sits down to eat," "you take out meat from the bison's body and roast it on fire . . . and a delicious well-balanced meal is served and everyone gets his share."[111]

Leisure and family are foremost in many of these social dreams and, as we will see, encompass both a relaxed social structure and a larger dream of economy based on "natural" evaluations of value. As Sargent has noted, the subset of mythic utopias in literature that, like the Paleo diet, look "to the past of the human race" are portrayed as "achieved without human effort. They are a gift of nature or the gods."[112] Indeed, the diets emphasize how nature bestows an effortless economy, claiming, "Life was more leisurely and less stressful, the human bodies were naturally fit" in caveman times.[113] Many dieters prefer the term "play out" to work out, as Paleo "playful and primal movement" exercise is reframed as a leisurely, fun way to express the body's natural desire to move.[114]

Some diets venerate hard work even as they promise cave-like leisure, often couched in the language of social cohesion of the original Paleo tribes. "They worked hard, but had ample time for leisure activities," acknowledges the 2001 *The Origin Diet.* "During their extended 'weekends,'" the story continues, "they became artists, painting caves with some of the world's finest pictures. They made elaborate jewelry to adorn their bodies. They sculpted flutes, played music and danced at parties."[115] *The Origin Diet* describes the familial intimacy of hunter-gatherer society, remembering how their "lives centered around family and community" and "elders were honored for their wisdom" by children sitting around "the campfire at night to hear stories."[116] A Paleo cookbook similarly promotes its "home-hearty" food that "harkens back to when families' [*sic*] took care of each other and ate their meals together."[117] *The Paleo Solution: The Original Human Diet* from 2010 combines comradeship and leisure, describing human ancestors as "early to bed, early to rise, and lots of adventure. . . . They had a strong social network, a sense of belonging, variety in their work and, really, not that much drudgery."[118]

Before promising that "weight loss just so happens to be a side effect of health and vitality," *Living Paleo for Dummies* paints an even more vivid picture: "So how did our ancestors live? They enjoyed a balanced life of working, playing, relaxing, and worshipping. . . . The kids laughed, played, and sang by the fire, and adults enjoyed conversation as they made plans for the next day. They felt closeness to one another and everyone had purpose."[119]

Passages like these suggest how many Paleo diets do not simply seek to recapture the caveman's health but the entire healthful worldview that produced such community, leisure, and beauty.

THE BODY UTOPIA AND RECALIBRATING
THE PLEASURES OF PAUCITY

But, as one diet asks, "What does this history mean to you?"[120] As Eaton *et al.* put it, "Who are we? Where do we come from?"[121] How does the body recapture its essential Paleolithic nature? We must turn to the body to recognize the story's bearing on the practice, the book on the body, or the myth on the manual. The "original human diet" offers an education of instinct and a deliberate, guided return to an intuitive sense of the body and its needs. Since the diet authors claim "the modern commercial world is leading our natural animal instincts astray—tempting us, teasing us, ensnaring us," the diet promises to repair the "damage to our innate sense of what's right for us."[122] Put another way, "the main 'trick' is to retrain your body; teach it to become more instinctive."[123]

In the 1975 *Stone Age Diet*, Voegtlin distinguishes between hunger and appetite, a distinction that continues to serve the Paleo community. Voegtlin claims that hunger is a purely "physiological mechanism," but appetite is an "acquired social endowment, a *conditioned* reflex."[124] Voegtlin and his colleagues promise that caveman diets bypass the construct of appetite so the dieter can recognize hunger and, once again, eat intuitively. For the "one million or so years before [man] began to acquire the doubtful assets of civilization," Voegtlin writes, "it is certain that nature also gave him a similar innate wisdom to choose foods best suited for his digestive tract."[125] After regaining true hunger, the dieter will naturally appease hunger with "whole" or "real" foods, effortlessly discerning what is *good* from what is *valuable*.

The dietetic utopia can be compared to the older "body utopias" characteristic of the Bakhtinian carnival or Land of Cockaygne. Pieter Bruegel the Elder's 1567 painting *The Land of Cockaigne* (Figure 1.4) best depicts the mythical land of plenty, troubling the celebration of unrestrained feasting by issuing a not-so-subtle comic warning about the aftermath of eating and drinking. Three bloated peasants lay helpless to finish an impossibly large banquet of sausages, cakes, meats, pies, and cheeses. A sliced

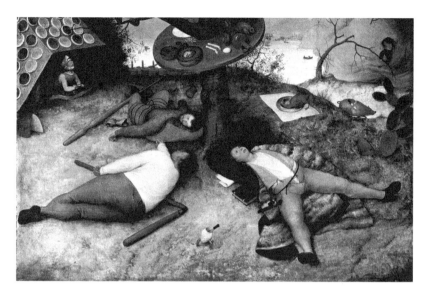

FIGURE 1.4. Pieter Bruegel the Elder's 1567 painting *The Land of Cockaigne* is a classic representation of the mythical land of plenty. Satirizing the aftermath of a feast, Bruegel paints peasants suffering the consequences of overindulgence in food and drink.

pig and half-eaten egg scamper by the prostrate figures, somehow taunting the peasants with their failure to finish the feast. The dietetic body utopia, on the other hand, venerates the restrained appetite and the regulated body by redefining pleasure; as the 2013 *Cavewomen Don't Get Fat* promises, Paleo foods offer a "calming, sustained sense of satisfaction," not the rash rush of a binge.[126] Likewise, *The Paleo Weight Loss Plan* claims that "once you've made the switch" to natural foods, an "entire pizza, a gallon of ice cream" will no longer taste delicious.[127]

Robert Fogarty notes that, in some ways, moderns already live in the Land of Cockaygne. In a 2005 *Antioch Review* editorial, he supports historian Herman Pleij's observation that, "by medieval standards, modern day Europe represents in many respects the realization of Cockaygne: fast food is available at all hours, as are climatic control, free sex, unemployment benefits, and plastic surgery that seemingly prolongs youth."[128] For Fogarty and Pleij, this modern fast-food world is less utopian cornucopia than dystopian glut, reviving older American notions of the distinctions between prohibition and temperance. However, the "world turned upside down" logic of this land of contraries still applies to contemporary utopian foodways.[129]

As Brenda Garrett notes, the word "Cockaygne" comes from the Latin *co-quina* (cooking), and "abundant and easy food" characterized many early utopian tales, often born from hardship.[130] Just as privation once produced the Land of Plenty, of "plenty of food and drink," now the Land of Plenty is producing fantasies of paucity.[131]

Both utopias—medieval abandon and modern restraint—are particularly appealing to the poor. Class distinctions still persist in utopian foodways: like the underfed peasant, the overfed poor today illustrate, at least stereotypically, the enduring relationship between body size and poverty. Ironically, the rich build immunity to this disease of affluence with tennis clubs and expensive salads, while cheap fast food and little leisure time dispose the poor to obesity. The Paleo diet still maps onto the Land of Cockaygne, however, in its reputation for expensiveness. Grass-fed meats, organic produce, raw nuts all rack up the grocery bill, many complain, but diet authors compare the cost of Paleo foods to later medical expenses. "Is it more expensive?" asked the *EasyPaleo* blog. "Yes, real foods will cost you more than fake foods," but Paleo foods mean "saving yourself from the inevitable medications, supplements, and even hospital bills that are looming in your future."[132]

The sensuous pleasures of food, so dramatized in the Land of Cockaygne or Bakhtin's carnival, are also reconceptualized in the caveman diet as tricks of wily industrial food production.[133] "Foods in flashy wrappers are attractive, sweet and tempting," cautions the 2013 *Paleo Diet*.[134] Extreme "foods that are sweet, salty, full of refined sugar, chemicals, and artificial flavors" lead only to "cheap food thrills," warns the 1985 *Dr. Berger's Immune Power Diet*.[135] Loren Cordain blames the "starchy gut bombs" of "artificial foods laced with unnatural combinations of fat, carbohydrates, salt, and sugar" for making "Americans the fattest people on earth."[136] Or as Walter Voegtlin expounds: "Our foods are chemically preserved, sweetened, colored, and flavored; they are canned, dehydrated, frozen, pasteurized, Fletcherized, fortified, ground, juiced, instantized, Osterized, precooked, prepackaged, puréed, pickled, salted, strained, and swallowed whole."[137] These methods of preparation dupe the body into craving fake flavors—extremes of salty, sweet, or, that sneaky blend of both, the Snickers bar.

Industrial food production has curdled the land of milk and honey. "The food industry is a multibillion dollar machine . . . full of addictively fake foods," warns the 2013 *77 Ways to Reshape Your Life*, "but you need to ask yourself 'Would this food be available to a cave man?'"[138] If not, chances are the modern food will dupe the body into mistaking deliciousness for goodness. Since humans are so easily hoodwinked by artificial flavors, the diets suggest that the traditional body utopias of abandon no longer work in the modern world. Rather than relishing an abundance of delights, the dieter would wind up binging on Doritos and Diet Coke.

Only natural foods can reteach the palate to recognize value; in Cordain's words, dieters must welcome the "return of your palate as Mother Nature always intended it to be."[139] With an educated palate, the body—not the industrial food system or the larger economy—determines value for itself. Cordain explains the process, assuring the dieter, "As you gradually wean yourself from salty, sugary, and starchy foods, your taste buds will become attuned to the subtle flavors and textures of wonderful real foods."[140] He describes them as "real, unadulterated foods."[141] In his cookbook, Cordain claims that "with the Paleo Diet, a fresh strawberry becomes exquisitely sweet and just right, whereas a fancy chocolate becomes too sweet—an artificial adulteration of the real thing."[142] The 1999 *NeanderThin* promises that, "in time, your sensitivity to natural sugar will increase to the point that raw fruit and small amounts of honey will totally satisfy any desire for sweets that you may have."[143]

Foods become "real," or, perhaps, decommodified, when the palate develops sensitivity to whole foods. These "evolutionary" or real foods gain value—not from their position in the economy or fetishization of the labor process—but from their relationship to the human body. The stomach biologizes the value of foods; for example, *The Everything Paleolithic Diet Book* reevaluates berries for their ability to lower blood pressure, not for their extreme flavors or cost per pound.[144] The dieter, then, learns to use instinctual corporeal recognition of foods that are *good.* Taste is educated away from both reckless delights and stripped of the social construction of value.

In this move to redefine pleasure by recalibrating the palate, we see that the calculated hungers of the diet are not sadistic pleasures. More is at stake in the reformulation of the body utopia from one of plenty to one of paucity; pleasure is actually reinterpreted as a reevaluation of quality and goodness. As Etta Madden and Martha Finch observe, utopian groups often use foodways to promise a future in "which human beings are 'saved' by learning to slow down, develop taste memories, experience true pleasure."[145]

This vision of the restrained body utopia is typical of the alternative food movement: slow foods, urban farming, farmers' markets, even Michelle Obama's victory gardens are cloaked in the rhetoric of restrained, moderated, and educated desires. As Madden and Finch note, slow food practitioners "defend 'quiet material pleasures' as the only effective antidote to the 'universal folly of the Fast Life.'"[146] Further, as Ruth Levitas has shown, the "education of desire is part of the process of allowing the abstract elements of utopia to be gradually replaced by the concrete" and, in very real terms, the education of the palate in the body literalizes the abstract elements of the Paleo utopia.[147] By the biological redefinition of pleasure itself, the body of the Paleo dieter is recast as receptive to only "true" or "real" pleasures which transform those reckless gratifications of Bakhtinian abandon into contemporary dietetic restraint.

MAYBE, ONE DAY: THE CAVEMAN DIET AND THE DIALECTICS OF UTOPIA

"Is this you?" *Dr. Gundry's Diet Evolution* asks readers. "Your skin is clear and unwrinkled, your slim body moves with ease and grace, and you're blessed with strength, stamina, and good health."[148] Did the diet "help you become a happier and kinder person," as the 2013 *Cavewomen Don't Get Fat* promises?[149] Or did it restore the Paleolithic world of family, intimacy, and belonging that Eaton *et al.* describe? Or, as they later ask, "Is it possible, then, to emulate the past?"[150]

In a word: no.

"Possibility and failure will forever be joined at the hip," Joseph Winters has argued in his study of utopia. "Hope and promise, no matter how radical, cannot escape the indelible human realities of death, suffering, and discord," and utopian projects "incorporate a sense of the tragic quality of existence."[151] Cavemen dieters aspire for ancient health but do so tragically, accepting that they can never revive what has always already been lost. "Unless the wooly mammoth is magically resurrected, it would be impractical, if not impossible" to eat as did our Paleolithic ancestors, the *Alpha Male Challenge* admits.[152] "You will not be scavenging meat from other predators. But, your shopping cart may be filled differently," *The Foundation Diet* continues, compromising the grand view of history to the contents of a shopping cart.[153] Rather, moderns can only learn from prehistoric habits and apply these lessons to their lives. We can't go back, the authors ultimately concede, but we can always still try by eating olive oil, walking barefoot, and dreaming of the past.

One Paleo dieter told me in an interview, after trying dozens of diets and embarking on a new one yet again, "You still think 'maybe,' you just think 'maybe'—maybe I can, maybe one day, maybe it will work this time."[154] Others share this optimism, but nearly all the forty-five million American dieters fail to lose weight or ward off weight regain.[155] Why try and fail, and try again, if failure is nearly certain? The answer, of course, lies in the extraordinary power of hope to enrich the imagination and give meaning to the world. The final failure of the caveman diet suggests that our hopes may be deferred by the diet, but they are never defeated; we are never perfect but forever perfectible.

In the end, then, the caveman diet is less concerned with losing weight than enlisting the body to strive toward a more ideal world. This is what makes the caveman diet a utopia. We need, however unattainable, the social dreams of original goodness and faith in the future, all bound in Sargent's utopian dialectic of hope and failure. "Risen apes or fallen angels," *The Paleo Manifesto* concludes, "we walk tall with eyes forward—one foot firmly planted on the ground of what we are, the other reaching into the future of what we can become."[156] And though we aspire for this future, the present pivots on that same firmly planted metonym of the foot. It is this foot—that banal, bodily thing—that reminds us of the cavemen we come from and the world we hope to create.

2 ⩗ DEVOTIONAL DIETS AND THE AMERICAN EDEN

T HE 2006 *HALLELUJAH Diet* opens with familiar words: "*In the beginning...*"[1] Hundreds of Christian weight loss diets published in the United States since the 1950s have continued that story: beginning in an Edenic world, falling into disease and obesity, and promising a return to that Edenic ideal if only Americans would improve their diets and ways of life. Devotional diets retell this familiar story—the narrative backbone of the Western world—that is at once the story of the Fall of Man and the fall of a once-blessed nation. In the tradition of the jeremiad, these diets condemn Americans for reneging on great promise even as they exhort Americans to change their way of life and improve the health of the nation. These diets are attempts at a grand new narrative of history and stand on the three-legged utopian dreams of a better self, a purer spirit, and a more perfect world.

Since the 1957 publication of Charlie Shedd's *Pray Your Weight Away*, devotional weight loss diets (also called Christian or Eden diets) have sold millions of copies to Christian and secular audiences alike.[2] In 1979, 1.4 million copies of Marie Chapian and Neva Coyle's *Free to Be Thin* were purchased.[3] In 2004, 2.5 million copies of *The Maker's Diet* were sold.[4] Approximately 15,000 congregants of Saddleback Church followed Rick Warren's bestselling *The Daniel Plan* in 2012 and lost a combined 250,000 pounds.[5] The last decade boomed with church-based diet programs such as *Firm Believer, Bod4God, WholyFit, Body Temple Wellness,* and *Body Gospel*.[6] The book titles speak a thousand words: *More of Jesus, Less of Me* (1976); *Help Lord—The Devil Wants Me Fat!* (1977); *Greater Health God's Way* (1984); *Adam and Eve Weren't Fat* (1999); *Diets Don't Work . . . But Jesus Does!* (2007); and, of course, the many punny *Garden of Eating* or *Garden of Eatin'* diets.[7]

Rising obesity rates might explain the appeal of Christian diet books.[8] Since the late 1990s, public health experts have found, regardless of socioeconomic status, religious Christians have some of the highest obesity rates in the country.[9] By the early 2000s, these findings were nearly irrefutable.[10] Doctors and sociologists offer different explanations for this disparity. Some argue that eating is an "acceptable vice" in a religious culture that discourages smoking and drinking.[11] Others believe the causal relationship could be reversed, suggesting that a church provides a "religious haven" for overweight people who feel alienated from mainstream American culture.[12] Still others have suggested that church participation—Sunday dinners, potlucks, and church suppers—itself contributes to obesity.

The obesity epidemic might have added a sense of urgency to Christian diets. Perhaps the culture of American health-consciousness, coupled with political efforts such as Michelle Obama's Let's Move program or alternative food activism, suggests their appeal. Or maybe the public weight loss of high-profile leaders like Rick Warren (who lost sixty-five pounds in 2011) inspired the growth in Christian faith-based diets.[13] These trends can, possibly, describe how these books soared to Christian bestseller lists over the last twenty years.

Yet these obesity trends cannot *explain* why these books tell the stories they tell. The need is real—weight control is a pressing Christian issue— but the diet book narratives are imaginative and complex. However important the political and epidemiological context, it is similarly important to listen to the stories the primary texts tell about contemporary America.

Interwoven in each diet book is a philosophical critique of modern America. These are stories about modernity, about time and pleasure, Western diet and Western sin, chastising Americans for their ill health and urging them to repent and reform the American way of life. Bitterly, dolorously, these texts imagine an earlier moment—in Eden, most often—in which sensuousness was holy, instinct was immediate, the body naturally craved good foods, and the concept of time had not yet been invented. Devotional diets are not just isolated Christian texts but actually suggest how Americans more broadly have conceptualized the effects of modern life on their physical—and spiritual—health.

This chapter contributes two main arguments to the discussion of food, religion, and the body in American scholarship today. First, my research contradicts the scholarly consensus on the legacy of Puritan asceticism in contemporary Christian diets by showing how these diets create a model of holy, sensuous pleasures. Food can be beautiful, the appetite pleasurable, and deliciousness divine in many of these diets. Devotional diets attempt to establish a seemingly natural relationship between instinct and time that uses the body's God-given or inborn instincts to gauge true pleasure when satisfied by true hunger. The promise here is that the immediacy of instinct, outside the bounds of time, recaptures the holiness of pleasure in the palate as an instinctual expression of God's will. Dieters reject worldly or legalistic evaluations of good or bad foods, sidestepping the mind and consciousness to resurrect the holy instincts for health. This, in turn, revives a healthy, timeless, universal model of Adam and Eve. And so these diets promise to teach what cannot be taught, to escape the bounds of mortality and trade history for eternity, to relearn instinct, and to undo the Fall.

Second, this chapter will demonstrate that, since the early 2000s, Christian diet books began considering obesity to be a collective—not individual—sin in the tradition of the American jeremiad. Contemporary books depart from religious dietary laws, dietary admonitions against the sins of gluttony and sloth; they are also very different from nearly all devotional diets published before the 2000s. Instead, most contemporary Christian diet books reconsider ill health to be an indiscriminate epidemic, infecting us all equally, with shared origins and a common cure. American landscape and body intertwine in this story about the divine in the body and the divine in the land, using the materiality of each to undo the Adamic curse of mortal bodies and barren environment. Eden is imagined as a real place, recalled by fruits and vegetables; however, eating holy foods does more than reignite God-given instincts. Holy foods also materialize the divine relationship between earth and body, nation and self, the grand enterprise of the New World and the American Adam. Earth and body, nation and self are made with the same material, mediated through the holy foods that meet God's highest standards. In this way, Edenic diet narratives judge the nation by its people's health and sickness, rethinking the success of a civilization in material terms of fat and thin.

Together, these two arguments indicate that Christian diet books published since the early 2000s offer a powerful critique of modernity that, in the tradition of the American jeremiad, interprets the meaning of America's past to urge reform and create a better future. Much like Paleo, precolonial, and detoxification diets, devotional diets pathologize the relationship between human health and modernity, interpreting modern diseases as biological expressions of social decline. Devotional diets, however, raise the stakes set forth by the other diets. Unlike the others, Christian weight loss plans fold the spirit into the larger claim of the diet genre on the whole—namely, that Americans today are fat, sick, and sad because our world is out of whack; Western civilization denies human nature and human needs; and disease is the inevitable cost of modern life.

This chapter also nuances the Freudian terms describing the instrumentality of self-control and willpower in the creation of the consciousness of the modern subject. If Freud considered sublimation and repression necessary to the success of civilization, then perhaps these Eden diets return to a world before knowledge to unearth bodily hungers as part of their broad critique of civilization. Devotional diets insist that dieters relinquish willpower to an ineffable hunger instinct embedded by God and stored in the human body. This material nostalgia for bodily instinct and timelessness works to move the mind out of the equation between innocence and knowledge. Instead, these diets attribute to the body the power to materialize a world that the mind can never re-create. Even at its most imaginative, the mind always mediates its own consciousness; nevertheless, these diets avow, the body can *make* a world that the mind cannot *think* into being. This Fall of Man philosophy points to how the diets provide new insight into popular interpretations of creationism and evolutionary theory. Many diets intertwine Adam and Eve into a longer, more complicated story about

ancestry, genetics, and the inheritance of physical traits. In a few rare in-
stances, less evolved primitive humans even predate Adam and Eve.

Eden diets also question the centrality of suffering to diet—a claim made
by much of food and American studies scholarship on the subject. Scholars
have inserted diets into American traditions of puritanical self-denial, inur-
ing themselves to the nuances of pleasure and joy offered by the texts themselves. Peter Stearns has called American Christian diet cultures "rigorous,
requiring too much punishment and denial," tracing weight loss diets today
to the enduring "American strain of moralism and self-sacrifice."[14] Harvey
Levenstein argues that twentieth-century American health food-faddism
is a product of the "residual Puritanism of the American middle class." He
reasons that "a culture that for hundreds of years encouraged people to feel
guilty about self-indulgence" could easily believe that "good taste—that is,
pleasure—is the worst guide to healthy eating."[15] Observers have also compared group weigh-ins to processionals and the pre-indulgence litany of
complaints—"The Calories, My God!"—to now be as "regular and ritualized as the saying of grace."[16]

Feminist scholars have argued that contemporary beauty ideals grew
from the secularization of Christian suffering. Joan Jacobs Brumberg argues
a 1922 diet book was "among the first to articulate the new secular credo
of physical denial: modern women suffered to be beautiful (thin) rather
than pious."[17] Michelle Lelwica suggests that suffering and self-denial are
still central to secular femininity, arguing that "the legacy of Eve is still
being repeated conceptually in contemporary Western culture" and "the
idea that women must suffer for beauty has supplanted (and perhaps incorporated) the belief that women must suffer to be holy."[18] More generally, Paul Campos condemns "our whole diet culture [which] is ultimately
about fear, and self-loathing, and endless dissatisfaction."[19] These scholars
do more than slot contemporary Christian diets into traditions of suffering
and actually suggest that Christian self-denial animates even the most secular contemporary American concepts of health.[20]

The history of Christianity also reveals how women used food depriva-
tion to reclaim control.[21] Brumberg's masterful history of anorexia examines
how female fasting upheld the holiness of the abstinent body, especially linking food refusal to virginal purity.[22] Other scholars have shown how female
food refusal was a method to transcend the "misogynist equation between
sin and flesh."[23] Amanda Porterfield argues that female mystics starved

themselves to "sacralize their humanity by identifying it with Christ's" and "consented to the belief that their nature as women was inherently sinful by punishing their bodies and by glorifying the suffering."[24] Food refusal was "physical suffering to transform the female body," another scholar notes, and the emaciated body was offered as proof of that suffering.[25]

R. Marie Griffith questions this secularization narrative in her careful analysis of religion in American weight loss culture. Dieting is too often cast as the secular sequel of an increasingly irreligious society, invoked as a metaphor to describe the "salvation of slimness" that "surfaces as the secularized 'sin' of overeating."[26] As Griffith expertly shows, American diets aren't simply an offshoot of puritanical self-discipline and they are not secular forms of older religious rituals such as confession or fasting. Rather, Christian leaders actively contributed to the American diet culture, creating a persuasive religious basis for American diets, both at large and specifically Christian. These leaders have pushed secular and religious concerns from spiritual to bodily purity. Building off Griffith's work, sociologists Samantha Kwan and Christine Sheikh have noted that Christian dieting itself actively resists secularization by adapting mainstream diet culture to "solidify a collective Christian identity" and "live a uniquely Christian life."[27] In the broad sweep of the secularization narrative across diet culture, most scholars have failed to notice the actual practices of Christian dieting which often contradict mainstream weight loss practices.

Many earlier Christian diet books villainized food, equating pleasure with sinful lust and fattening foods with defilement. With the onset of the obesity epidemic, however, most Christian diets broke with the secularization of suffering framework. By contrast, contemporary Christian diet books use imaginative, lush language to dwell on the sensuousness of taste and pleasure. Descriptions of beautiful apples, emerald cabbages, rich-tasting treats that tingle the tongue abound. Some unabashedly describe, as does the 2012 *Holy Eating*, the gratifying "pleasures of smelling, tasting, and chewing" or, in *The Eden Diet*, the "taste [of] sensual pleasure."[28] They do not call for the denial of pleasure but rather the selective enjoyment of God's embodied pleasures. Pleasure is still strictly regulated by skipping over the mind entirely and directly appealing to the instinct of the body which, in turn, is an unmediated manifestation of God's evaluation of the goodness of foods. Some dieters even pray for the ability to enjoy these pleasures: *God, I see from Your Word that You gave me vegetables and fruits as food. I want what You want for me. . . . Change my palate, Lord, and help me begin to eat vegetables and fruits. I will do it by faith, God. But help me enjoy it."*[29]

The fundamental structure of the diet—as a plan of food restriction—might bear its debt to Christian traditions of self-denial, but the language and tone of diets published since the early 2000s legitimize the pleasures of food. "We should not feel guilty when we eat delicious food," Rita Hancock states in *The Eden Diet.* Even "rich, delicious foods" are good if the dieter, for example, "eats the éclair to the glory of God."[30] Compare Hancock's éclair to an earlier éclair described in the 1979 diet *Free to Be Thin:* "You wouldn't want to eat a hair, a roach, or a rat, but that eclair or those greasy french fries may be just as defiling."[31] Griffith explains how this type of Christian diet invoked disgust by calling rich, fattening foods filthy and unclean.[32] One minister condemned delicious foods by explaining: "If you enjoy what you're eating, chances are that it's bad for you. Your menu has been formulated by the devil to tempt you to ruin."[33] By contrast, a 2013 diet explained that "God made eating sustaining, delicious, and pleasurable because God is all these things and more."[34] Though a few diets still condemn eating as devilish temptation, the broad history of devotional diets reveals that something big happened in the thirty years between *Free to Be Thin*'s 1979 rat-like éclair and *The Eden Diet*'s 2009 delicious treat.

CHRISTIAN WEIGHT LOSS LITERATURE: AN OVERVIEW

The first commercial Christian weight loss book was published in 1957 by the Presbyterian minister Charlie Shedd.[35] Titled *Pray Your Weight Away,* the book outlined a severely restricted diet that accused overweight Americans of ruining God's temple. "When God first dreamed you into creation, there weren't one hundred pounds of excess avoirdupois hanging around your belt," Shedd writes.[36] Fatness is a sin, Shedd argues, averring, "We fatties are the only people on earth who can weigh our sin." Like many diet authors after him, Shedd inspired his disciples with stories of his personal weight loss. "Before" and "after" photographs of Shedd on the back cover of *Pray Your Weight Away* illustrated the efficacy of his plan.

Three years later, Deborah Pierce published *I Prayed Myself Slim* when she was just twenty-two years old. Pierce weighed over 200 pounds during her miserable adolescence, taunted by the other children as "fatty, fatty, two-by-four, can't get through the kitchen door."[37] Despite many attempts on commercial diet plans, Pierce only lost weight when she acknowledged her sin of gluttony. *I Prayed Myself Slim* outlined a punishing 1,000-calorie diet, describing how Pierce lost 100 pounds by skipping lunch and dinner for two glasses of water and prayer.

Shedd continued to publish diet books into the 1970s, most notably *The Fat Is in Your Head* in 1972, which leapt up to the list of National Religious Bestsellers and stayed a bestseller for two years.[38] In 1975, Frances Hunter wrote *God's Answer to Fat: Loose It!* and another evangelist, Ann Thomas, wrote *God's Answer to Overeating*.[39] The *Los Angeles Times* reviewed Hunter's book and, with three printings in six months, religious booksellers reported that copies flew off the shelves.[40] Perhaps the most visible of Christian diet leaders, Gwen Shamblin founded her church-based Weigh Down Workshop, Inc., in 1986. By Shamblin's own account, 30,000 churches implemented her workshop and, later, she sold over a million copies of her 1997 *The Weigh Down Diet*.[41]

Since the 1970s, the number of Christian weight loss diets have more than tripled, crossing over into more mainstream diet culture with the 1979 publication of Marie Chapian and Neva Coyle's *Free to Be Thin*, which sold 1.4 million copies worldwide. To borrow Griffith's words, Christian diet literature went from a "trickle to a torrent" in the late 1960s and early 70s.[42] This "torrent" of 1970s devotional diets clearly precipitated the even bigger flood of Christian weight loss books today.

Yet the trends in devotional diets have not been continuous or predictable. Analysis of commercial Christian weight loss books since the 1960s reveals a marked shift around the early 2000s. Before then, most diet book authors considered overweight indicative of some characteristic social, moral, or religious deficit. After the early 2000s, Christian diets began reinterpreting obesity as a national failing and offering a historically specific condemnation of American disease-causing culture. This collective approach challenges scholarly belief in a nineteenth-century shift from "the modern Western body understood as a collective product of inscription" toward "a personal projection of the self."[43]

Alarming epidemic obesity rates may have also helped shift blame from the individual toward the nation.[44] Compare Shedd's two books, for example: in 1957, Shedd railed on fatties who could weigh their sin. In 1972, Shedd mentions sin only once, and that's in a footnote. Most likely, Shedd softened his tone because, as he explains in the first sentence of his 1972 *The Fat Is in Your Head*, "Are you one of the overweight millions living life in quiet desperation?" If so, "then you've got company." Shedd reports that "too many pounds is the nation's number one health problem."[45] Despite the milder appeal to the Christian community of "heavies," Shedd still blames "fatties" for "flabby thinking." He called one "huge junior-high boy" a "pitiful creature."[46] No matter how common obesity had become in the United States, Shedd still faulted the individual.

Since the late 1990s and early 2000s these diet books aligned with the now-common explanation for the American obesity epidemic that points to the American way of life. Since more than one-third of all American adults qualify as obese and two out of three are considered overweight or obese, government policies have explained the epidemic as a broadly American problem.[47] Devotional diets, the Food and Drug Administration (FDA), and policy initiatives all recommend vegetables, whole grains, and exercise; all three warn against high-fat, high-calorie processed foods and sedentary lifestyles. Both Christian diets and government guidelines sometimes get specific, blaming screen time, vending machines, television, beauty ideals, plastic surgery, and so on for the nation's poor health.

Christian diets rejected explanations of gluttony, sloth, or other individual ills for obesity and instead blamed American culture. "Sickness comes from the collection of garbage in our SAD, Standard American Diet," George Malkmus argues.[48] *Jesus' Diet for All the World* calls it the "'The Great American Food Machine' [which] consists primarily of either life-debilitation or life-destroying foods."[49] Even the American dream was fair game. A 2002 diet called "eating one of America's favorite pastimes," because the "fundamentals of the American Dream are expressed in a desire for *more* and *bigger*."[50] The three opening words of Rick Warren's *The Daniel Plan* are *"Wow! Everybody's FAT!"*[51] Ted Haggard, author of the 2005 *The Jerusalem Diet*, observes that, in a roomful of leading pastors, "*Everyone* in the room was overweight." In fact, "pastors are the single fattest group of people I know!"[52] To fight the obesity "epidemic in our society," the 2004 *Fit for God* insists, "We need to stop focusing on our personal goals and issues and start thinking collectively and corporately." Collective problems require a social cure, however, and in the next paragraph, *Fit for God* explains that "people were created to work together for the common good of all mankind."[53]

Devotional diets also cast a wide net by using universalizing, gender-neutral language, appealing to men and women dieters alike by invoking comprehensive ideas of a Christian congregation or community. Evangelical diet book authorship even skews male.[54] Some devotional diets also include non-Christians, explaining that Eden was a shared experience and everyone, whether they acknowledge it or not, descends from Adam and Eve. The first two sentences of one Jesus diet begins: "You don't have to be Christian to benefit from the Jesus diet. After all, Jesus was not a Christian."[55] In turn, some evangelicals have suggested the diets might help spread Christianity or, at least, encourage dieters to rededicate their "life to Christ."[56] In fact, *The Serpent Beguiled Me and I Ate* appeals to Jews, Christians, and Americans who are "not members of an organized church," by explaining that everyone participates in the "historical drama of eating," with "origins deep within the Judeo-Christian tradition."[57]

Christian diets might share arguments with American diets and government advice at large, but the differences are telling. Devotional diets make plain the religious tenor of dieting culture, refine concepts of pleasure, and challenge assumptions about creationist or evolutionary thinking. For that reason, the bibliography is composed of strictly Christian weight loss texts published in the last few decades, with particular attention to the diets of Reverend George Malkmus, Rita Hancock, and Jordan Rubin. As originators of high-profile diets with diverse religious and medical backgrounds, these authors provide fresh insight into accounts of human origins, whether strictly creationist or loosely evolutionary.[58]

"TRAGEDY TO TRIUMPH": EDEN DIETS AS REINVIGORATIONS OF THE JEREMIAD

The story devotional diets most often tell is a familiar one: in Eden or an Edenic world, the human race was naturally healthy and beautiful but humans fell into disease and despair. Today, obesity and modern disease are ruining our nation's health and impending doom can only be averted if Americans radically change their diets and ways of life. While many devotional diets explicitly follow the Adam and Eve story, others less obviously deliver the same narrative by holding up images of the natural world against current corrupted society. Whether or not explicitly Edenic, devotional diets follow the narrative arc of the jeremiad as they lament the loss of an original ideal, warn of society's impending downfall, and exhort Americans to change their ways and return to that original ideal. It is unsurprising that devotional diets narrate what is, arguably, the most familiar literary narrative in the Western world. More important for a deeper understanding, however, is how devotional diets use the individual obese body to channel larger concerns about the success or failure of America and, even more broadly, the human race and its endeavors to make for itself a civilization.

Devotional diets often share mainstream millennial rhetoric warning that obesity and diet-related disease will cripple the American people. Media regularly report that obesity ruins children's self-esteem, American sex life, and military performance, or, more generally, "how obesity threatens America's future."[59] Even some diet invectives pale against government warnings. In 2003, Surgeon General Richard Carmona called obesity an urgent and grave "health crisis affecting every state, every city, every community, and every school across our great nation."[60] Devotional diets do more than replicate conventional doomsday predictions; they toggle between fear and hope, and are themselves practical plans designed to spur action. The rhetoric in *The Hallelujah Diet* or *The Maker's Diet* are jeremiads that push Americans to quick and practical action: to eat and live in only the ways prescribed by the diet.

Devotional diets situate today's obese Americans in a longer account of human history that begins with an Edenic ideal. But one major difference divides them: some diets strictly adhere to the 6,000-year-old creationist account of human origins and some incorporate evolutionary thinking or some sense of man's primate forefathers. The second category of evolutionarily inclined diets begins with Adam and Eve and then meanders through the invention of stone tools, agriculture, and food processing techniques, and finally culminates in the unhappy state of obesity and sickness in America today. Both types of longer narratives—strictly creationist and more flexibly evolutionary—justify close analysis.

This chapter first looks at the creationist account in George Malkmus's 2006 *The Hallelujah Diet* and then, for contrast, at the flexibly evolutionary religious account of human history in Jordan Rubin's 2004 *The Maker's Diet*. Even to a casual reader, the differences between Malkmus's *The Hallelujah Diet* and Rubin's bestselling *The Maker's Diet* are striking. Malkmus insists that only raw, vegan foods sustain life while Rubin furiously rejects the stereotype of the "wimpy vegetarian health guru" and urges Americans to eat more red meat and saturated fat.[61] Rubin uses a modified evolutionary synthesis to recommend "primitive" foods while Malkmus refuses evolution wholesale, insisting the earth is 6,000 years old. For every oat biscuit and lentil recipe in *The Hallelujah Diet*, Rubin has recipes for rich desserts and red meats. Rubin's recipes are defiant, rich concoctions: the mocha mousse is made with beef gelatin and heavy cream, and one 748-calorie lamb dish combines the triple whammy of red meat, sugar, and port wine in the same meal.

On the face of it, Rubin and Malkmus share little in common. However, their texts follow the same narrative formula of the jeremiad, offer the same critique of American civilization, and enjoin Americans to make similar changes to their diets and ways of life. In fact, the petty differences between oat biscuits and mocha mousses indicate the enduring power of the underlying jeremiac narrative. The profound similarities between *The Maker's Diet* and *The Hallelujah Diet* suggest that these texts are not (and have never been) about lamb or lentils; rather, these are big and powerful stories about sickness and health, about God and man, and the human race and civilization.

The Hallelujah Diet follows two decades of Malkmus's work preaching the miracles of natural living after curing his colon cancer with raw fruits and vegetables. In 1994, he and his wife Rhonda established a health retreat, called Back to the Garden Ministries, in Tennessee.[62] He published *God's Way to Ultimate Health: A Common Sense Guide for Eliminating Sickness through Nutrition* in 1995 and *Why Christians Get Sick* in 1996. Malkmus himself estimates that, since its 2006 publication, *The Hallelujah Diet* has helped more than two million dieters lose weight and regain health.[63] Malkmus's company owns millions in property and pays sixty full-time employees.[64] Malkmus cross-promotes his nutritional supplements and health retreats with Hallelujah Acres Publishing, which has produced spin-offs such as Rhonda Malkmus's *Salad Dressings for Life* (2002) and *Hallelujah Holiday Recipes from God's Garden* (2006).

The Hallelujah Diet tells a typical account of the Eden diet story—beginning with the beginning of the world and ending not with death but the promise of eternal health and beauty and joy. Malkmus narrates a 6,000-year history of human development and refutes evolutionary thinking, exclaiming that we must "turn from man's feeble attempts to explain the origin of *life* without God, through a process called evolution, and turn to the Bible, where we learn the true origin of *life!*"[65] Even as he discounts evolution, Malkmus's vegan diet is a plan entrenched in beliefs about human history and the dangers of modernity. False wisdom, science, "frankenfoods," and the Standard American Diet all figure into this new account of human history that still begins in Eden but falls, precipitously, with American civilization.

Malkmus gives example after example of the sick made well and the weak made strong. His wife, Rhonda, dropped ten dress sizes after losing eighty pounds on the diet.[66] Malkmus insists God and the Bible showed him the way to cure his cancer through nutrition. After finding a baseball-sized tumor, Malkmus decided not to undergo chemotherapy for colon cancer. Instead, he went on a diet of "raw fruits, raw vegetables, and one to two quarts a day of freshly extracted, raw vegetable juice."[67] His cancer disappeared. He regained the energy of a twenty-year-old. He no longer suffered from allergies and sinus problems. His pimples vanished. His eyesight improved. "Every other physical problem I had been experiencing also disappeared!" he exclaimed. "*Totally healed!*"[68]

"Humanity has lost its way," Malkmus begins. Science, the Age of Enlightenment, the ivory tower, and civilization itself has corrupted our health, according to Malkmus. He explains that "our civilization has stitched together a chemistry experiment involving chemically fertilized food, chemically sprayed to kill the bugs, chemically preserved . . . 'Franken-foods.'" Since the "Age of Enlightenment [and] modern science," Malkmus mourns, "the modern views of nutrition and health became corrupt."[69]

Malkmus combines conventionally historical and religious histories to warn of impending doom. In an invective colored by italics and exclamation marks, Malkmus foresees the fat getting fatter, the weak growing weaker, and the entire country crippled by obesity. "Ah, the American dream!" he ironizes, after sketching a "day in the life" of an average American. As Malkmus describes it, Americans live in misery and anger. We stress over impossible deadlines, yell at our children, sleep terribly, and our lives are spent "constantly running to beat the clock." Poor diet is responsible for this misery, accounting not only for obesity and general malaise, but also road rage, child abuse, anxiety, and schizophrenia. Given this state of the nation, Malkmus exclaims, "It's no wonder the illness and death statistics are so staggering!"

However far we have fallen, Malkmus assures dieters that they can always change their health. "Even though we might reside in the Modern Babylon, we still have the freedom to choose our own menus," he promises.[70] *The Hallelujah Diet* will recover the "simplicity of God's system [that] became lost" with the development of modern civilization. In terms of individual health, as well, Malkmus declares his optimism. "But there is *hope!*—even if the deterioration of the body cells is quite advanced." Hope is possible because the Hallelujah Diet provides the "proper fuel for miracles." Malkmus exhorts his readers to submit themselves to the Hallelujah Diet, which uses an eating plan to anchor a critique of American civilization.

At its most basic, the Hallelujah Diet is vegan, mostly raw, and low in calories. Malkmus prescribes daily doses of the living enzymatic BarleyMax supplement (sold on Malkmus's website for $5 an ounce) and three daily glasses of vegetable juice.[71] Malkmus classifies all animal products as "dead" foods and warns that, "regarding cooking, there is a very fine line between *life* and *death* in terms of temperature."[72] "God designed us to be foragers," he stresses, and Adam and Eve did not cook what they foraged in the Garden of Eden. Recipes include directions for oat biscuits, lentils, and faux Spanish "rice" made with onions and grated cauliflower.

Food is only one part of the program. Malkmus insists Americans wear their seatbelts, drive slowly, turn off the TV, share their hearts, slow down, and stress less. He cautions, ominously, "There is one last element of doom that you should avoid at all costs—negative and destructive thoughts."[73] Allegedly, these practices and foods (and expensive supplements) cure disease because they resurrect the embedded healthfulness—God's self-healing immune system—in our ancient bodies. Once these instincts are rediscovered, dieters will develop a sense of pleasure to calculate what foods are good and godly and what foods are bad and man-made. This is the promise of return: when Hallelujah dieters return "to the very diet that God, our Creator gave Adam, and through Adam to all mankind some 6,000 years ago, their bodies will receive healing."[74]

By evoking a magnificent, healthful past, Malkmus urges Americans to return and re-create an Edenic world long lost. Malkmus offers a deep-historical vision of life, reflecting that we can "trace our *life* back to God! And as a result of the offspring of those two God-created human beings, Adam and Eve, human *life* has been handed down generation after generation, for the past 6,000 years, until ultimately you and I were born."[75]

Situated in this holy history, the calamities of the obesity epidemic can be reinterpreted not as certain doom but as an opportunity to change, repent, and work toward reform. In this way, the body acts as a fulcrum and a fossil—shifting the force between past and future while it demonstrates the tenacity of the human race across history and through time.

Jordan Rubin wrote *The Maker's Diet* in 2004, nearly ten years after his brush with nearly a dozen life-threatening illnesses. As Rubin tells the story, he was *"literally starving to death"* and even naturopathic medicines worsened his arthritis, diabetes, chronic fatigue, hair loss, anemia, and Crohn's colitis. Only 114 pounds at his sickest, Rubin despaired until he discovered God's health plan in the Bible. Today at a healthy and fit 185 pounds, Rubin believes that "the Maker has given me a program for vibrant health based on his Word." He has dedicated his life to "telling the world the truth that will set them free."[76]

Rubin has built an empire out of God's health plan which, as he promises, helps dieters lose weight while curing everything from colds and cancer to Crohn's disease and candida. In 2004 and 2005, *The Maker's Diet* spent forty-seven weeks on *The New York Times* bestseller list. In 2009, Rubin watered down his religious rhetoric with *The Maker's Diet for Weight Loss*, but his fiery 2004 version is still the most successful. As of 2014, Rubin's publisher counted 2.5 million copies of *The Maker's Diet* in print.[77] Before the Maker's Diet series, Rubin published *Patient Heal Thyself* in 2003, a similar plan for "overcoming incurable illness."[78] Rubin repackaged much of *Patient Heal Thyself* into *The Maker's Diet*, and, later, he and his wife, Nicki Rubin, collaborated on two health books for women and children. Rubin's dietary supplement parent company, Garden of Life, made over $40 million in sales in 2003.[79] The Federal Trade Commission sued Rubin for deceptive advertising in 2006, but the lawsuit did little to damage Rubin's reputation.[80]

"You hear the alarm screeching in your ear as you peer at the clock . . . in disgust," Jordan Rubin begins *The Maker's Diet*. Like Malkmus, Rubin uses the same second-person perspective to illustrate a "day in the life" of a typical American: a life dogged by aches and sluggishness, fatness and stress. "You look in the mirror" and see "dark circles underneath bloodshot eyes," feel twinges of guilt that your children are overweight and asthmatic, worry because your mother is arthritic, and mourn for "your father [who] died last year of a massive heart attack." It is a painful and scary depiction of an average American life, but, Rubin assures his readers, "If this story sounds a lot like yours, *you are not alone*." Ill health is a shared problem because, as Rubin writes, "the state of our health as a nation is worse than ever before."[81]

The Maker's Diet follows the same jeremiac arc as *The Hallelujah Diet* and nearly all Eden diets of this period. Rubin first bemoans the current state of civilized nutrition and then interprets modern disease as a sign of national failing, warning of imminent doom, tempered with the assurance *"we can change."*[82] Like the others, he believes modern life has created a modern body racked by false hungers, trapped in a fallen world, and overwhelmed by sadness, sickness, and stress. Rubin compares our modern age to an earlier, better stage of the human race, complaining that "in our era, we have allowed food to become our idol" and "most modern men and women have strayed far from the Creator's foods." American diet and food industry practices are at fault but Rubin takes his invective further by blaming the American way of thinking. "In our promiscuous society, we say *yes* to virtually every whim and desire of our palate, resulting in a national dilemma of becoming overweight, sedentary, and an increasingly sick population," he writes.[83] Even worse, America has provoked the "globesity" epidemic. In an ironic twist of global leadership, Rubin writes, "Like an Olympic flag bearer, the American contingent is leading the globesity parade."[84] Doom gives way to hope, however; if dieters follow *The Maker's Diet*, they will "pull themselves out of the grip of disease and enter the promised land of health."[85]

Citing early twentieth-century studies of the isolated, primitive peoples of Kitava and Gabon, Rubin speculates about prelapsarian nutrition in Eden to argue for the broadly diseased properties of civilization itself—not simply civilized nutrition. Like most followers of primitivism, Rubin uses the term "primitive" to describe more of a constellation of cultural and religious ideals rather than a precise period (however mythic) on the timeline of human history. For Rubin, primitive nutrition is muddy, somehow slotted into the mixed-up chronology of cavemen, precolonial peoples, and Adam and Eve. Primitive humans or hominoids rarely figure into creationist accounts of Adam and Eve's fall from grace, but Rubin uses both "our primitive ancestors" and God's original humans as models for contemporary nutritional and life advice.[86]

After a subsection titled "The Hidden Cost of Being Thoroughly Modern," Rubin exclaims, "We must leave behind our disease-producing diets and lifestyle and return to our Creator's dietary guidelines, as incorporated in the Maker's Diet!" Rubin writes that "the wisdom in our physiology and biochemistry cry out for a primitive, biblical diet," even though our diet has been so deprived of the foods "designed by the Creator and eaten by our ancestors." Primitive societies were healthy *until they switched to modern diets.*" Generalizing from these examples, Rubin states, "Modern civilization has managed to infiltrate the culture of many of these once-isolated societies and . . . this transition from primitive diets to modern diets has brought *deadly consequences.*"[87]

Rubin draws heavily from the work of Weston Price, an American dentist who published extensively in the 1930s and 40s on the nutritional superiority and healthfulness of primitive life. In *The Maker's Diet*, Rubin calls Price "one of his nutritional heroes," summarizing Price's work in *The Maker's Diet* with subheadings titled "Primitive Diets Produce Beautiful Teeth, Strong Bodies" and "Modern Diets Produce Physical Degeneration."[88] Price's studies were rife with racist speculation and unpalatable politics but, today, Price is known primarily for his argument that high-carbohydrate Western diets caused poor dental health and the diseases of civilization.

Rubin describes a theory of human development that seems, at first glance, to replicate the Paleolithic diet narrative of the originally healthy caveman. Like Paleo dieters, Rubin believes agriculture brought about modern disease. "The scientific analysis of skeletal and dental remains of primitive societies from the past were stronger, bigger, and healthier than those who lived after that societal change," he elaborates.[89] Rubin lays out a specific timeline, drawing from archaeological evidence that demonstrates the decline of human health around 1150 AD in North America. Yet Rubin uses the language of God's original design and the holiness of embodied instinct to add religious righteousness to narratives most often told as secular, even Darwinian. Though Rubin's conflation of God's original design and primitive nutrition might seem blasphemous or misguided, the logic of Rubin's argument is sound. He is more generally advocating for a return to a past—any past—not so much to recapture Eden but to renounce modern life.

Although Eden has seldom been reconciled with evolutionary narratives, Rubin shares in a tradition merging caveman-like elements with depictions of Adam and Eve after the Fall. Before Darwin, most common was the depiction of the expulsion as a painful, final condemnation. Thomas Cole's 1828 *Expulsion from the Garden of Eden* (Figure 2.1) beautifully

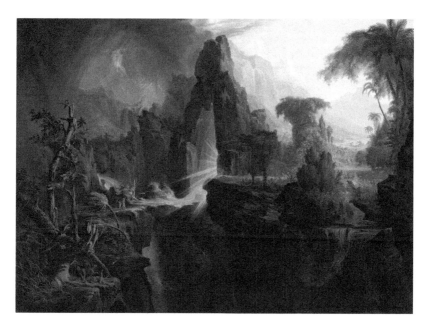

FIGURE 2.1. Hudson River School artist Thomas Cole's famous rendition of Adam and Eve in *Expulsion from the Garden of Eden*. Adam and Eve are physically shut out from the Garden by shards of light and clothed only in beige, nondescript wrappings. Thomas Cole, *Expulsion from the Garden of Eden*, 1828, Museum of Fine Arts, Boston.

represents the finality of God's decision: Adam and Eve literally shut out by the shards of light expelling them forever from the timeless Garden. Cole guides the eye from timelessness into time by way of two waterfalls. In the Garden, a gentle, wispy waterfall circles back on itself, while, in the fallen world, a violent plunge of water races down a gorge, gathering force as it falls.[90]

After Darwin, some artists occasionally rendered Adam and Eve with primitive or Paleolithic traits. One 1908 illustrated guide to the Bible depicts Adam and Eve hunched, forlorn as they make their downcast departure stage-right from the Garden of Eden (Figure 2.2). Yet this artist clothes Adam and Eve in animal skins, dressing Adam in a spotted cheetah toga, a stereotypical representation of caveman apparel at the time. Angels still watch over Adam and Eve as they depart and, as the text explains, "Accompanying the curse upon man came the divine promise of redemption."[91]

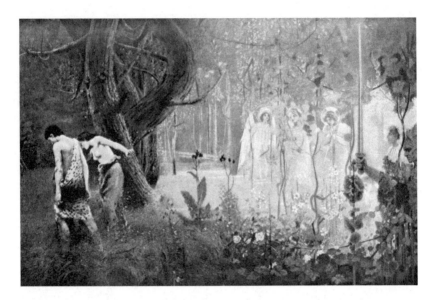

FIGURE 2.2. Artist Abbey Altson paints Adam and Eve clothed in animal skins stereo-typical of representations of caveman apparel in a 1908 illustrated guide to the Bible. Although Adam and Eve are rarely depicted as primitive versions of mankind, some Garden of Eden diets adopt and recommend elements of Paleo or primitive nutrition.

Paleolithic traits situate Adam and Eve into a narrative of possible progress rather than expelled and forever doomed to sin. Unlike traditional representations of Adam and Eve condemned for eternity, Paleolithic Adam and Eve look more like immature versions of mankind's modern self. Devotional dieters more generously interpret the expulsion, in a way especially relevant to the project of the diet, by recasting Adam and Eve as primitives capable of improvement. Paleolithic Adam and Eve present more opportunities for reform on the linear narrative of evolutionary progress.

By calling obesity a national crisis, Malkmus, Rubin, and their contemporaries depart from earlier texts that explained obesity with the rhetoric of gluttony, sloth, and other sins. Post-1990s diets also invoke the language of political action or collective responsibility for American fitness on the whole; as Rick Warren insists, "The Daniel Plan is not a book. It's a movement."[92]

In the early 1950s, historian Perry Miller demonstrated how the jeremiad helped shape New England society in the late seventeenth century, conflating the spiritual project of the Puritans' "errand in the wilderness" with the religious founding of the United States.[93] As a pronouncement of doom and failure, the jeremiad incited New Englanders to renew their spiritual commitment to God's call to create a holy nation. Sacvan Bercovitch elaborated in his landmark 1978 book, *The American Jeremiad*, showing how the jeremiad continued to shape American concepts of the self well into the nineteenth century. Unlike older European jeremiads, the American jeremiad fused secular and sacred history similar to the way that Rubin conflates primitive Native American societies and the sacred blessing of nutritional purity. God and nation mixed in the jeremiad which, as Bercovitch shows, "united nationality and universality, civic and spiritual selfhood, secular and redemptive history, the country's past and paradise to be, in a single synthetic ideal."[94]

Devotional diets operate on the same structure of jeremiac time: of past, of fall, of paradise promised. Bercovitch shows how the jeremiad could "simultaneously lament a declension and celebrate a national dream" to renew American commitment to its own foundational national story.[95] Eden diets mourn for a healthy past (before SAD, in an Edenic America), berate Americans for their fall (the obesity epidemic), and reinvigorate the commitment to a national dream (happiness and its pursuit). Obesity endangers the whole national project. As Charles Stanley, the senior pastor of the First Baptist Church in Atlanta, warns in the foreword to Rubin's book, "Our nation's health is at an all-time low." Rubin reiterates Stanley's claim a few pages later, noting that "the state of our health as a nation is worse than ever before." Widespread obesity leads to diabetes, cancer, and heart disease, Rubin fears, suggesting that many Americans only escape cancer because fatal heart attacks claim their lives first.

Jeremiads like these are gentler than their predecessors. Even though "it seems our very existence as a species is threatened if we don't change," Rubin offers "good news for you: *we can change*. We can redirect our own health destiny."[96] Rubin's first chapter is titled "From Tragedy to Triumph," and tragedy to triumph could just as well summarize the narrative arc that depicts an original standard, narrates the fall from that standard, and, finally, reenvisions and promises the ideal. Today, while these diets admit that America may have gone astray, Americans are still infinitely perfectible and can try (and try again) to achieve the ideal.

RETHINKING PLEASURE, OR, EDEN IS A REAL PLACE

If not the obese, who is to blame for the American obesity epidemic? Why and how has America fallen so far? Eden diets answer these questions with two subtle arguments. First, they blame the American food industry and SAD for deluging the palate with false pleasures and, second, they blame modern structures of time for overruling the natural timetables of hunger unique to each body and appetite. Together, these engineered flavors and unnatural clocks blind and deafen the body to its own God-given instincts toward healthfulness.

Most obviously, modern foods have overruled God-given instincts toward the true pleasures of healthy, holy foods. "Techno-foods," overcivilized (and unnatural) appetites, and processed "hyperpalatable" foods deceive Americans and pit their bodies against the engineered flavors of modern industry. However, the food industry not only offers "frankenfood" tastes that trick the palate but has also lied to Americans about the healthfulness of their foods. As Philip and Agnes Maynard explain in *The Jesus Diet*, the "food industry . . . processes [food] in such a way that it leads people to put on weight" and also, perhaps worse, misinforms Americans by labeling sugary, fiber-deprived foods as "'fat-free' and 'low-fat.'"

Instinct and nature are set into stark relief against industrialization, technology, and, most broadly, the concepts of modernity and progress. "The quintessential fast-food trio of 'burger, fries and Coke' perfectly illustrates the food industry's ability to capitalize on our most instinctual taste preferences," Rachel Marie Stone explains. Modern foods are "endlessly engineered, tested and re-tested for 'hyperpalatability,' making them addictive as well as irresistible."[97] Even our brains are defenseless against these tricks, Rick Warren argues, writing that our "brain chemistry is hijacked by hyper-processed, hyper-palatable, hyper-addictive foods."[98] Jordan Rubin explains that "we stray far from God's design with an array of techno-foods rich in empty calories."[99] The biblical *Get Thin, Stay Thin* program explains how worldly distinctions of value overrule God-given hunger instincts and labeling like "right and wrong, good and bad inflames our sinful nature."[100] However, "God knows what is needed in our bodies and by our instincts lead[s] us to proper nutrition," writes James Creed in his 2003 book of God's answers.[101]

Or, as *Look Great, Feel Great* summarizes, "we get corrupted by the foods made by men in laboratories and factories" when we deviate from "the foods that come from God."[102] Rubin makes a similar claim in *The Maker's Diet*, explaining that prepackaged foods might "reassure us they are 'enriched with 12 vitamins' or that they are '100 percent natural'" but these claims are misleading at best. "The unfortunate truth is," Rubin claims, that these foods, which "overload our bodies with adulterated fats and refined sugars," have strayed very far from God's original cuisine.[103]

If these modern pleasures are unhealthy and unholy, the dieter's task is to learn to distinguish between fake, modern pleasures and true, Edenic pleasures. The diets teach this distinction by separating out natural hunger from cultural appetite, explaining that natural, holy foods satisfy true hunger while unnatural, modern foods appeal only to the appetite.[104] In their claims to reclaim true hunger, these dietetic Edens promise to reteach what cannot be taught—to educate instinct, to redo history, and undo the Fall. Materiality in body and land is central to these longings for unmediated instinct. As the following will show, the diets educate a disciplined body to restrict—naturally—its experience of pleasure by toggling between a divine landscape that produces food and the healthful body that takes pleasure from that same food. Pleasure is sanctioned because it is God's pleasure, mediated through true hunger and compelled by instinct.

Eden is described as a real place and a cornucopia of real pleasures, replete with the delights that actual earthly landscapes provide—puffy clouds, red apples, tangy berries. Rachel Marie Stone notes in her diet book, "Scripture describes the Garden of Eden as a place of abundant, beautiful, delicious food."[105] Far more than other diets, Eden diets describe the aesthetics of food, often by asking dieters to imagine a material vision of the Garden of Eden. "Picture in your mind a feast of foods that were put here on earth by God—a diet full of nuts, whole grains, beautiful and colorful fruits, and vegetables," *The Diet of Eden* asks its readers.[106] Another diet tells readers, "Imagine Adam seeing for the first time . . . the huge fruit trees, fresh springs of water, and multitude of flowers."[107] Or, as Malkmus summarizes in *The Hallelujah Diet*, Eden is a place of beauty, with "sight, touch, smell, and taste."[108] Malkmus describes a real, sensuous landscape abounding with delicious foods, a beautiful and warm place populated by healthy physical bodies. "God gave Adam and Eve, and all of mankind who would follow, the ideal way to nourish their marvelous physical bodies," Malkmus claims, creating a theory not in the abstract but in the material.[109]

Aesthetic pleasures are also invoked far more often in devotional diets than in other types of diet books; the beauty of the human body and foods are praised for manifesting God's divine intent. "God wants to make you beautiful," Marie Chapian and Neva Coyle assure dieters in their revised 1994 *Free to Be Thin*, praising foods such as a "beautiful plate of raw vegetables without dressing" and "six to eight glasses of beautiful water" for their splendor. *Free to Be Thin* dieters should show their appreciation by saying, "Praise God, I'm eating beautiful, healthy food . . . a beautiful six-ounce serving of swordfish."[110] Pointing to the larger shift away from self-denial, all three of these descriptions of beauty—of swordfish, water, and raw vegetables—are noticeably absent from *Free to Be Thin*'s original 1979 publication. After substituting God-pleasing foods for forbidden foods by following the 2009 *The Day Begins with Christ* plan, you can "give in to your indulgences and live and eat like God wants us to."[111]

One testimonial written by Malkmus's cowriter, Stowe Shockey, draws out the health-giving pleasures of holy foods—foods that miraculously arrested the progress of her precancerous cervical cells and her husband's heart disease. She describes these delicious, holy foods in loving detail in her section titled "Back to the Garden." Reflecting on her home-grown gazpacho ingredients, Shockey watches giant squashes wave to her in the breezes of her garden, calling, "*Look at me!*" Those beautiful yellow plants were the "most delicious squash and zucchini I ever had the pleasure of eating." "I could hardly wait for them to finish," Shockey said of her cabbages, because "nothing cools me down like coleslaw made from those emerald globes." The tomatoes were equally delightful, described as "tall and vibrantly green, while the pale little balls decorating them still waited for the earth and sun to make them rosy red."[112]

Deliciousness overwhelms Shockey. While sipping her gazpacho, Shockey "paused, savoring the flavor, imagining the living enzymes causing the tingling sensation on my tongue." Other forms of deliciousness overpower her whole being: "With each bite, I sank a little deeper in bliss. But curiosity aroused me, for there were other tastes to try." These "rich-tasting treats" not only satisfied her hearty appetite but were also "simply delicious."[113] Bliss, satisfaction, richness, arousal, and deliciousness: language like this characterizes most Eden diet discussions of holy, healing, and weight-loss-inducing foods.[114] These diets plainly contradict the scholarly idea that Christian weight loss today fits into an old religious tradition of

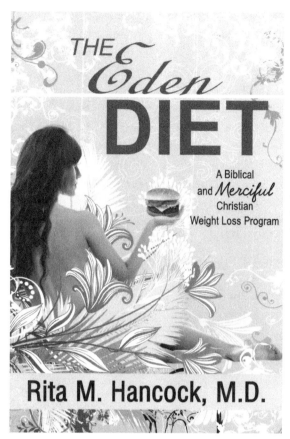

FIGURE 2.3. *The Eden Diet* book cover from 2008 depicts a nearly nude Eve holding a cheeseburger in her right hand. The diet suggests that all foods—even cheeseburgers—are permissible because all foods originate in God's Eden. Rita Hancock, *The Eden Diet: A Biblical and Merciful Christian Weight Loss Program* (n.p.: Personalized Fitness Products, 2008).

self-denial. In fact, Haggard directly confronts this tradition, promising that his *Jerusalem Diet* will teach dieters to "relax and enjoy the food you like without nagging guilt."[115] And Hancock is still clearer about God's gift of pleasure, even incorporating modern foods into her version of the Edenic diet (Figure 2.3).

She asks her readers, "God allows us sensual pleasure in other ways without guilt, so why should we feel guilty when we eat in the way he intended?" Comparing food to a beautiful sunset or symphony, Hancock asks, "Why do we feel guilty when we taste sensual pleasure?"[116]

Rachel Marie Stone seconds the question in her 2013 *Eat with Joy: Redeeming God's Gift of Food*, asking, "And why did God make eating so pleasurable?"[117] Subtracting "the biological explanation—food is pleasurable so that we'll eat it, mere incentive for survival," Stone believes "that God made eating sustaining, delicious and pleasurable because God is all those things and more." Indeed, much of her book advocates for the redemption of pleasure, insisting, "We should revel in—not be ashamed of!—our enjoyment of the simple pleasures of smelling, tasting and chewing."[118]

Malkmus, Hancock, Stone, and many other contemporary Christian diet authors legitimize these pleasures because, in this formulation, God gave man the instincts to detect holy pleasure. In turn, God imbued food with the pleasures of taste and satiety: apples with tang, strawberries with sweet, wheat with chewy, grainy texture. The hunger for God is a real hunger, satisfied by real pleasures of a real place—Eden. In the tradition of the American sublime landscape, Eden bridges between earthly pleasures and divine presence.

These holy pleasures—tang, sweet, salt—make sense in the Edenic portrayal of the American landscape. The divine vision of the American landscape mixes a view of bodily and national health, echoing long-standing myths and symbols of the Jeffersonian farmer, the divine sanction of the colonial project, and the therapeutic promise of the land.[119] Malkmus explains, "Can't you just envision the brilliant blue sky, with the puffy white clouds, and the crystal-clear atmosphere, along with all those brilliantly colored foods just waiting and ready to be plucked?" He wants his readers to imagine "man's beautiful home" covered "with beautiful, brilliant, red apples that are shimmering and glimmering in the sunlight."[120] In this dietetic, leisurely Eden, dieters can eat in God's presence and take pleasure from bodily delights.

Edenic nature opposes culture and civilization most clearly in the distinction between hunger and appetite. Nearly all Eden diets admonish Americans for following their conditioned, cultural appetites rather than their natural, inborn instincts toward hunger. As Shannon Tanner explains in her 2007 *Diets Don't Work . . . But Jesus Does!*, "God placed in us a natural system to regulate hunger, which in turn will regulate and maintain our true and desired weight."[121] This untaught instinctual system resides in all people but, Tanner regrets, many Americans are cut off from God's natural regulatory systems. "Most overweight people eat from *appetite* and have lost sensitivity to the sensation and regulatory direction of true physical hunger," marking the difference between "*true physical hunger* and *false hunger or appetite.*"[122]

Lysa TerKeurst's 2011 *Made to Crave: Satisfying Your Deepest Desire with God, Not Food* explains the fuzzy distinction between spiritual and sensuous hungers. Our cravings are real and good, she insists, but misguided: the hunger for junk foods is simply a hunger for God. "Eve craved what she focused on" and didn't consult Adam before eating the apple, TerKeurst clarifies. Much like how Eve's "cravings displaced God" and brought about the Fall of Man, TerKeurst admits that "I craved food more than I craved God."[123] Tanner explains that appetite creates "lean spirits and bulging bodies" because we have lost our understanding that "the root of our hunger [is] the empty cry of our souls which longs for intimacy with a loving, gracious, and all-knowing God."[124] The *Hungry for Jesus* forum promises freedom from unhealthy food behaviors by "choosing God—not food behaviors—to satisfy our innermost needs."[125]

In the 1980s, Gwen Shamblin's Weigh Down Workshops pinpointed the confusion of "physical hunger and spiritual hunger" or, as she sometimes calls it, "*stomach hunger*, rather than *head hunger* (or *desire eating*)" as the cause for weight gain.[126] "Spiritual food," according to Shamblin, "should be food for the heart" but it is food nonetheless—food presented as delicious and satisfying, even if it pleases the spirit more than it does the palate. Spiritual hungers are confused for stomach hungers but both are legitimately sensuous. Cravings are real and the hunger for God is no less tangible than a hunger for salt or sweet or savory. "Natural God-designed foods" are delicious because they are healthy, *Faith and Fitness Magazine* reports, "for God so loved the world, He gave us sun-dried tomatoes, Honey-crisp apples," and other holy foods.[127] Dieters mistake appetite for hunger only because they have been duped by the food industry and modern ways of life—not because the dieters are sinners or gluttons.

Malkmus offers the most detailed explanations of instinct's role in ascertaining God's nutritional design. Malkmus explains, "God the Creator placed all the 'instincts' . . . so that man would naturally be drawn to those foods that contain the vital nutrients."[128] SAD and modern ways of life have overruled the hunger instinct so dieters no longer have access to the instincts which gauge the healthfulness of foods. In fact, SAD creates a cycle of toxic food addiction and "people confuse their addictive withdrawal symptoms with genuine appetite."[129] Withdrawal symptoms include headache, cramping, weakness, fatigue, or shakes which dieters interpret as hunger sensations. However, Malkmus argues, dieters must wait for hours until these symptoms subside and then they can experience true hunger.

With true hunger comes the ability to recognize God's handiwork in the pleasures of holy foods. God made healthy foods beautiful and they charm the eye as well as the tongue. Malkmus expounds, "Instinctively, we are attracted to the beauty, the smell, and ultimately the taste and texture of that appeal of the apple." Instinct translates into action, as Malkmus describes. "Instinctively, the man goes to the tree, plucks a beautiful apple from the tree, and instinctively takes a bite from that apple." Apple in hand, "Instinctively, we start chewing that bite of apple with the teeth God placed in the mouth at the time of man's creation." Instinct operates the teeth handed down directly from God and directs the grinding chew according to God's design. If we eat as did Adam and Eve, Malkmus swears that older instincts to glorify God will reawaken and dieters will relearn the instinct to choose healthy, holy foods.

Only instinctive digestion extracts value from these foods. Malkmus explains, "Instinctively, I take a bite of the carrot. Are the nutrients immediately available at cellular level? No! So instinctively . . . I start chewing it." After chewing, "I instinctively swallow it," and produce a pulp that "slides down the esophagus." Later, "dripping digestive juices" will release nutrients into the bloodstream.[130] In a kind of Marxist formulation, this carrot is the exact opposite of a commodity because the stomach biologizes the intrinsic value of carrots, not their cost per pound. In fact, the unmediated commerce between carrot and its value to the body can only be brokered by instinct, far from rational thought and even further from social relations. This carrot deviates from what Karl Marx described as the "commodity-form, and the value-relation of the products of labour within which it appears . . . have absolutely no connection with the physical nature of the commodity."[131] Labor is nowhere to be found in this precapitalist Edenic garden and, in fact, only the "physical nature" of the carrot determines its value.

Malkmus's story of human history hinges on the immutable human body. The indelibility of instinct—that kneejerk response to chew the carrot—is proof that God built us as he did Adam and Eve. Even in the twenty-first century, our memories are Adam and Eve's memories because our bodies are Adam and Eve's bodies. That sensual sense-memory of Eden resides within our bodies, ready to be awakened by the foods that are "shimmering and glimmering in the sunlight." Taste bypasses modern food addiction and shortcuts to the holy instincts of true hunger. Malkmus believes that imagining the Garden will "*jog your memory*, because there was a time when our ancestors knew that life comes from life."[132] Just as Proust's Madeline revived memories long buried, Malkmus swears that healthy food today will awaken our memories of that holy Garden. Our healthy God-designed diet might be instinctual, but Malkmus fears this instinct has been lost in the development of modern civilization. By reviving taste as an instinctive evaluation of foods, Malkmus claims that the body will relearn both its own needs and God's original design.

THE HOLY TIME OF THE BODY

Modern structures of time (when to eat) are second only to industrial foods (what to eat) for obscuring the God-given instincts that once, naturally, gauged the holiness and healthfulness of food. By postponing meals, dieters do much more than eat less; they sensitize their palates to the instincts of hunger and satisfaction and, in turn, desire and pleasure. "Why is God's timing and His 'food' best?" asks one diet.[133] Another explains: "As people learn to respond to their God given signals of hunger and fullness, and forego worldly legalistic food rules," then they can expect "lasting and eternal changes in" their "body, mind and spirit!"[134] Those signals of hunger and fullness can be revived in abiding by God's holy rhythms of the body. Dieters must be patient and listen for God to express his will, a message of hunger mediated by the natural instincts of the body. "*Lord, help me to remember that Your timing is perfect. Amen*," another prayer implores.[135] Only by waiting for God's hunger signals, arising from instinct, can dieters take true pleasure from the satisfaction of true hunger.

"Do not be afraid to wait a few hours for hunger," Shamblin instructs her readers in the *Weigh Down Diet*, sharpening the distinction between the lower intestine rumbles of "trying to digest the last supper" and the authentic stomach growl of "true physiological hunger."[136] Jesus fasted for forty days, Shamblin recalls, and dieters should learn to appreciate the natural feelings of hunger growls and other stomach signals. Every dieter's body rhythms are different. "Some people have had to wait for three hours; some have had to wait a day and a half," but all, Shamblin writes, must "look for a small, empty feeling or growl" to "relearn how to feed the stomach." In *Diets Don't Work ... But Jesus Does!* Tanner explains the benefits of waiting in detail: "Waiting on God's timing and provision go hand in hand with the natural principle of waiting on true hunger. . . . Yet when I wait on God's natural timing for my body, not only will I enjoy the food that much more, but I can relish in the freedom of waiting. Waiting requires trust, love and faith. Are you willing to wait on God?"[137]

In *The Eden Diet*, Hancock elaborates that only by waiting can dieters skip consciousness and regain connection to the internal instincts of true hunger. In a subsection titled *"Let Waiting Be Your Offering,"* dieters are assured that "waiting shows how much we trust the internal signals he gave us [and] how we love and respect the bodies he gave us." She reasons that one should "consider it an act of worship to wait, and thank God for the discipline that lets you do it." Waiting might require discipline, but dieters can always rely on God's support to rediscover the truth of hunger pangs and Hancock promises that, if dieters "quote Scripture, pray, and meditate, you will be able to resist the temptation to eat prematurely."

But when the urge strikes, Hancock encourages the dieter to eat and eat well.[138] She believes undue waiting is dangerous. "Don't go hungry for too long," Hancock warns, because once dieters "identify" and "appreciate" hunger pangs, they are "ready to eat the food [they] desire." Hunger pangs are God's gift and Eden dieters should "realize that they are useful sensations given to you by a loving Creator who has your best interests in mind."

After waiting recovers the pangs of true hunger, Hancock explains how these instincts will reunite God to the body. In fact, Hancock believes that self-consciousness and knowledge hurt more than help our health. She explains:

> Even before Adam acquired self-consciousness at the Fall, his body would have been fully capable of taking care of itself. . . . If we break a bone, we grow it back together. And we do it without thinking. If we had to think about it, we'd probably mess it up. By intelligent design, your blueprints for healing and your blueprints for weight loss were hardwired into you in the beginning, and they are still accessible to you. In the case of healing from your obesity, you just have to learn how to relax your intellectual desire to control, submit your hunger pangs to God, and let the healing begin.

In Hancock's narrative, the hunger instinct bypasses the mind and communicates directly to the body. The mind can be dangerous, even, and pervert the hunger instinct embedded by God and since stored in the human body. By teaching dieters to appreciate and act on instinct, these diets attribute to the body the power to materialize a world that the self-conscious mind can never re-create. As a direct conduit between God and the world, the instinctual body can materialize a vision of nature and God that the mind cannot *think* into being.

In this concept of the body, waiting until true hunger clears the pathway between instinct and satisfaction allows God's time to reintegrate into the timetable of the body. God's time opposes the slotted timetables of modern life which, as Tanner describes, take away our "natural and instinctive" hungers. "Because of scheduled mealtimes and activities that revolve around food," Tanner explains, we have "learned a different pattern of eating by instead responding to appetite and not true physical hunger."[139] By resisting these scheduled mealtimes and instead waiting for God's timing to determine true hunger, dieters use a spiritual vision of instinctual time to overwhelm the false dictates of appetite. Holy time resituates the individual into a longer history that begins with Adam and Eve but persists, unchanged, in the timeless human body. History—that linear before and after—is redefined as an always-now through the shared material of the same body. God's design is at once original and simultaneous, directly communicated via the same instincts, the same stomach growl, the same rhythm of hunger and satiety, the same teeth God once put in the mouths of Adam and Eve. The diets create a seemingly natural relationship between instinct and time, using the body's inborn instincts to determine when hunger compels eating. Real hunger comes unmediated from the body, Hancock and others argue, and should be satisfied quickly because that satisfaction is God's will.

This praise of instinct challenges much of the current thinking about Christian attitudes toward the body, usually set by studies of sexuality, arguing that the church and biblical thinking attempt to intervene between biological urges and expressions of those urges. Sexual instincts are urges to be overcome outside of marriage but, with hunger, these urges must be heeded. While the instinct to have sex might be real and strong and nearly impossible to resist, it is forbidden outside of the divine institution of marriage—not when instinct compels. "Biologically, teenagers have raging hormones," *Why You Should Not Have Sex before Marriage* explains, and "the temptation for premarital sex is very real, physically."[140] Even though this instinct is embedded in God-given biology, the urge must be overruled by civilized, religious dictates of the church and society. Like hunger, the sexual drive is God-given and instinctual, but sexual urges can only be expressed at the proper time and with the proper partner: in marriage, with a husband or a wife.

Christian weight loss texts take the opposite view toward these biological desires. Hunger should be obeyed precisely because the instinct is so urgent and strong it cannot be resisted. The diets venerate untaught pleasures and rank God-given instincts as superior to the dictates of the church. In fact, the church and the day-to-day Christian lifestyle is *blamed* rather than praised for cultivating poor eating habits. "Potluck means bad luck," a 2000 diet puns, and breaking bread in fellowship now looks like "the church table is loaded with chocolate donuts, angel food cakes, apple pies, fried chicken dinners."[141] The 1979 diet book *Free to Be Thin* concurs, asking its readers, "How many Sunday school picnics have you gone on where you heaped your paper plate so high with food?"[142] Another diet leader put it wryly: "I haven't seen a fruit or salad bar [at church] yet."[143] Hunger is not externally sanctioned by religious life but is instead validated by God-given instinct expressed in the irresistible and "true" desire to eat. This "true hunger," according to Christian weight loss leaders such as Tanner, TerKeurst, and Creed, is a sign from God, transmitted through the instincts of the body, to eat, find pleasure, and feel satisfied.

THE FACTS AND FICTIONS OF THE OBESITY EPIDEMIC

Both in fact and in fiction, the obesity epidemic has become a collective concern, with common causes and common cures. Devotional diets lend themselves to the jeremiac form because obesity presents a unifying health epidemic. Rhetorically and generically, after that transition in the late 1990s or early 2000s, contemporary devotional diets exceeded the realm of self-help and individual concern about women, body image, food politics, or identity. These new diets are simply one part of the bigger, grander narratives about American disease that raise the questions that make the world worth thinking about: life and death, nature and culture, God and man, the success and failure of human civilization.

But theory and high thinking aside, we must return to the stories the texts tell about ourselves. What do the diets promise at the other end? Where is this after-and-before world of health and beauty? Dieters are necessarily vague because hope is an infinite horizon and, as Bercovitch writes, jeremiads work only because the American dream is a "'dream,' as prophecy" and never a realized goal. One representative from Hallelujah Acres told me, soon after following the Hallelujah Diet, "you start feeling good, feeling healthier, feeling better . . . just start feeling overall better." Some dieters might lose weight or cure their cancers, but everyone would "feel good, just better, overall just better."

Rick Warren's blockbuster *The Daniel Plan* elaborates. He explains the meaning of healthy eating and weight loss: "Real food has the power to give you your life back and more fully engage in the purpose for your life. The reason to do it is not to fit in your jeans or look good in a dress, but to be awake to the beauty and miracle of life, to be able to live with purpose, to love, serve, connect, and celebrate the gifts God has given you."[144] A step further, *The Jesus Diet* vows that "the contents of this book could save our contemporary world." The diet will "redeem us as individuals from a common destiny of disease and death. . . . [It is] the sure path to creative peace, to superb health and beauty, to an optimal abundance of joy in life."[145] Despite the hucksterism and moneymaking, mostly these messages are told truthfully, with sincerity and vision. Warren trusts in his diet because, partially, his message of hope *will* awaken Americans to the beauty and miracle of life. Even if the diets never work for weight loss, they work to enrich the imagination, to inspire change (however small), and offer hope for a better world.

This sentiment is most piercing in modest books, self-published by small-town pastors or full-time housewives. When Texan Barbra Sonnen-Hernandez, mother of two, fell sick and recovered from a rare disease, she was inspired to write the 2011 *The JESUS Diet: Taking the Weight off Your Soul.* If her readers are very sick, Sonnen-Hernandez reassures them that God gave them the foods to "live a longer, healthier, and happier life." Gently, she says that "it's more than the body. It is your soul that needs to be brought out in you; it's the buried treasure that reveals the precious gem that is you."[146]

She tells her readers to go to a full-length mirror. The reflection looking back might be overweight or unhappy, with an unflattering hairstyle, but, Sonnen-Hernandez writes, "You're not a failure; even though you're overweight, deep inside you're a beautiful person waiting to come out, and the world can't wait to see such beauty God has given us." Even though you are "weak and vulnerable . . . concerning your weight problem," Sonnen-Hernandez gently assures her readers in poetic form: "Nothing will hurt me anymore/I have no problems that are a problem/I am sure of my life and the direction/It will go now/All things are possible/Because I found you/And you love me."[147]

Sonnen-Hernandez offers this sincere message of hope and love alongside recipes for tacos and summer salads. Her calorie chart outlines the benefits of raw vegetables: squash for the heart, bananas for blood pressure. This message of hope is just as real as the vitamin content of vegetables; one does not demean the other but, rather, together, this mix is both a plan and a promise. And the diet itself—that real, practical plan of squash and sugar-free lemonade—is what suggests why pessimism so often buckles before visions of hope.

3 ❧ PRIMITIVE DIETS AND THE "PARADISE PARADOX"

|N 1979, A study in *Diabetes Care* reported on the "disastrous health effects of westernization" in the Pacific Islands.[1] A 1991 medical report concluded, "For Samoans, modernization produces obesity."[2] By 1997, the International Diabetes Federation referred to diabetes as "a Western killer let loose in Paradise."[3] In 2007, a front-page headline in the *National Post* was still more blunt: "Obesity Epidemic Destroying Paradise."[4]

"Primitive" or "precontact" diets respond to fears like this by promising a return to Native diets before colonial contact. Primitive diets eschew industrial foods, cultivated cereals, foreign imports, and nonnative crops. In the wake of colonial encounter, many of these diets approach Native peoples as living specimens of a more healthful past who represent an earlier stage on the evolutionary timeline. The diets are sometimes called ancestral, traditional, indigenous, or primitive, but all are premised on the mismatch between modern life and ancient bodies. Or, as the Ancestral Health Society manifesto puts it, the ways modernity has "pushed our physiologies dangerously far from their adapted environments" has resulted in the "epidemic flood of illnesses collectively referred to as the diseases of civilization."[5]

Unlike Paleo or Eden dieters who follow a diet common to a shared human history, most primitive dieters separate people by different bloodlines or ancestries, arguing that some dieters are optimally adapted to certain points on the timeline of evolutionary development. Primitive dieters can be "Natives" themselves, distinguished by heritage, genetics, body shape, or blood type, or else outsiders looking to learn a lesson from colonial encounter. While some dieters locate the precolonial paradise by going back before the invention of fire (raw and living diets), others position original health before foreign crops were introduced or global trade brought in imports. All the diets are defined by contact—the moment in which a previously healthy race is brought into the modern world, introduced to contemporary foods, and made vulnerable to the diseases of civilization. After praising the meaty diet of the Inuits, Weston Price, an influential mid-twentieth-century American diet researcher, retold the story: "Like the Indian, the Eskimo thrived as long as he was not blighted by the touch of modern civilization, but with it, like all primitives, he withers and dies."[6]

Three groups of Native peoples have braced the American medical approach to precontact diet: Native Alaskans, Pacific Islanders, and, to a lesser extent, Native Americans. For the last hundred years, doctors, anthropologists, and self-styled experts have catalogued Native ways of life and promoted supposedly uncorrupted natural diets. By using the simple contrast of nature and culture, these studies of "primitive" life shore up an American identity as "civilized" by comparison. Primitive diet research also adds complexity to the concept of imperial nostalgia, showing how mourning a vanished race hides the fear that Westerners are next in line. Put another way, the diagnosis of dying primitives sounds the death knell for the human race.

Diets investigating all three Native foodways plumb the periphery of the nation and test the dangers of a deadly diet on the most vulnerable people. Of the three, however, only the Pacific Islands diet has ever crossed over into popular weight loss practice. For context, an overview of both Native

Alaskan and Native American diets provides insight into the special popularity of Pacific Islands weight loss. Until the 1940s, the high-protein meat-based Inuit diet fascinated researchers testing the role of vitamins and fat in proper diet. In his 1913 *My Life with the Eskimo*, the Arctic explorer and Harvard-trained anthropologist Vilhjalmur Stefansson (1879–1962) described his meaty diet heavy on caribou, wolf, squirrel, and boiled seal flipper. Stefansson returned to New York in 1928 and ran a high-profile diet experiment while hobnobbing with the intellectual elite and romancing the writer Fannie Hurst, who later wrote a captivating dieting memoir titled *No Food with My Meals*.[7] For his year-long experiment, Stefansson enthusiastically ate a high-fat diet exclusively of meat—beef, lamb, veal, pork, and chicken—and the experiment is still cited today as medical proof of the safety of an all-meat diet.

But the Inuit diet never caught on in popular practice and remained a faraway romance of precontact life. As Susan Yager noted, meat consumption during the 1930s had declined due to increased beef prices, changing tastes, and diet advice. Stefansson's gruesome descriptions of meat may also have hurt his cause. For a public still reeling from gory descriptions of meatpacking in Upton Sinclair's 1906 *The Jungle*, Stefansson's instructions on how to roast caribou head from "the base of the tongue to the center of the brain" or make "cold seal blood" soup may have been less than palatable.[8] When compared to the Pacific Island diets, the Arctic also has a very different cachet in the American imagination. Up against *The Tropical Diet* plan of fruit salad and creamy tropical cocktails, caribou brain is a tough sell.

Despite a rich history of medical research, a Native American diet has also never crossed over into weight loss circles. When this flurry of medical and anthropological exploration into diet began, many assumed that few Native American tribes remained untouched. As far back as 1839, diet reformer Sylvester Graham relied on secondhand observations made by Plymouth colonists that the noble, hardy Indians ate the "plainest and simplest forms of food," mainly maize, groundnuts, and acorns. By the time Graham wrote, he already mourned the "noble race" who had been "treacherously robbed of [their] country, then cruelly exterminated as savages."[9] A hundred years later, in 1939, Weston Price also detailed the challenge of finding "original stock" Indians still "living in accordance with the tradition of their race" outside "the influence of the white man."[10] As Philip Deloria noted, the colonists celebrated Native Americans for their hunting prowess and colonists feasted on New World foods of savory meats and Indian drink in ritualized Tammany dinners.[11] Two centuries after these savory feasts, most Americans were no doubt aware that overhunting had decimated indigenous meat animals: the bison population shrank from an estimated sixty million bison before 1800 to under a thousand in 1880. Combined with a reputation for alcoholism, Native Americans must have seemed like unlikely candidates to inspire twentieth-century Americans looking to lose weight.

More recently, the Pima Indians of Arizona laid the foundation for modern diabetes research and inspired community health initiatives to replant native crops and revive older cooking techniques. A 1971 study found that half of all Pima Indians over age thirty-five had type 2 diabetes, the highest recorded diabetes prevalence in medical history.[12] Today, more Pima American children likely suffer from diabetes than any group of children in the world. Researchers have tracked these rates since the mid-1960s, generating a huge data set regularly mined by diabetes researchers from all over the world to better understand and prevent diabetes.[13] Given similarly epidemic rates, medical publications often categorize the Pima and Pacific Islanders together to show how rapid rates of modernization increase diabetes risk among genetically similar populations.[14] Since the late 1970s, diabetes research has cited these disparities to show how a "traditional lifestyle" protects against type 2 diabetes within indigenous populations.[15] In 2001, one *Journal of Internal Medicine* article observed that diabetes and obesity are the "devastating results of Western intrusion into the lives of traditional-living indigenous communities."[16]

All three of these discourses engage in what Renato Rosaldo aptly called "imperialist nostalgia," a complex feeling in which the "agents of colonialism long for the very forms of life they intentionally altered or destroyed." A feeling of "innocent yearning" conceals a "complicity with often brutal domination," he clarifies. Not only does yearning assuage troubled consciences but also, as Rosaldo explains, colonists use a static "savage society" as a "reference point for defining (the felicitous progress of) civilized identity."[17] A double-edged sadness, no matter how sincere, celebrates the success of the colonial endeavor. In this "dreamwork of imperialism," colonists wish away their own corrupting influence, yet look back to a static, timeless prehistory to measure the forward march of Western civilization.[18]

Imperialist nostalgia captures the sadness that imbues precontact diet, but misses the dread. It toughens the softer feelings of fear. Locked into precontact diets is the image of the obese Inuit or diabetic Hawaiian as a threat. The story told by white diet reformers often goes like this: your fall is not only our disgrace but also signals our demise. Natives are more vulnerable to the deadly American diet, but non-Native Americans are far from immune. After photographing "isolated and modernized Polynesians" in the 1930s, Weston Price reflected:

> Many of the island groups recognize that their races are doomed since they are melting away with degenerative diseases, chiefly tuberculosis. Their one overwhelming desire is that their race shall not die out. They know that something serious has happened since they have been touched by civilization. Surely our civilization is on trial both at home and abroad.[19]

Western disease had put civilization on trial and found it responsible. And the case of doomed island races proves that the first to fall will not be the last.

Nostalgia of this sort also colored British discussions of the healthy diets of Native peoples under their jurisdiction. The British regularly lauded the natural foods and agricultural methods of the traditional Indian diet during colonial rule.[20] Beginning in the 1920s, the British colonial physician Sir Robert McCarrison published his observations about the superior diet of Northern Indians. McCarrison described Northern Indians as a race "unsurpassed for perfection of physique and in freedom from disease," especially the stomach maladies so common among Westerners (ulcers, dyspepsia, appendicitis, some types of cancer). "The unsophisticated foodstuffs of nature is compatible with long life, continued vigor, and perfect physique," he commented in 1921, advocating for unsophisticated, undoctored food that we would now call whole foods.[21] His subsequent nutritional experiment with rats fed either on the Sikh diet or the working-class European diet confirmed that processed foods caused ill health.

As Harvey Levenstein documented, McCarrison soon inspired other British and American doctors to conjecture about the ills of modernity by praising remote peoples, in particular the healthy Hunza of modern-day Pakistan. The Hunza Valley already held significance for the British, who could "imagine an imperial vision in which remoteness stood as a sign of the vastness of the British Empire," as one scholar recently noted. Remoteness itself also stood against modernity, framing "an antimodernist discourse" that critiqued Western commerce, industry, science, and agriculture.[22] The 1936 *Wheel of Health: The Source of Long Life and Health among the Hunza*, authored by G. T. Wrench, also a British doctor, was an early blockbuster for American health publishing company Rodale Press and is still widely cited in diet books and organic farming manuals.

Though the British example and Native American and Alaskan diet research help provide context, Pacific Islands diet advice also merits special attention because, of the three, only the Pacific Islands has entered into popular weight loss diets. Only the Pacific Islands still retains its grip on the American imagination in diets, narrating the Fall of Man plot in the context of colonial encounter and portraying the main characters—Native Pacific Islanders—as bystanders in a historical drama about health and the consequences of colonialism.

American precontact Pacific Island diets can be traced to Sylvester Graham (1794–1851), James Salisbury (1823–1905), John Harvey Kellogg (1852–1943), and Weston Price (1870–1948), who all recommended diets drawn from peoples they considered primitive. All four men used indigenous diets as a yardstick to measure the American body, soul, and nation. Usually, America came up short. As religious health reformers, both Graham and Kellogg linked natural vegetarianism to sexual control. Salisbury endorsed meaty Native American diets to Americans ravaged by the Civil War and, with a type of salvage ethnography, Price and also Stefansson searched the world to document the diets of primitive peoples.

In 1837, Sylvester Graham praised the carbohydrate-heavy diets of Pacific Islanders for producing a fine and athletic race of modest, pleasant people. Graham described Islanders as tall, handsome, robust, with unruffled good humor and ivory-toothed smiles.[23] As Kyla Wazana Tompkins argued, Graham "vacillated between celebrating primitivism" and extolling the "civilized life" in America. By using Pacific Islanders as "examples of primitivism as living relics of the civilized world's prehistory," Graham built up the ideal American character as both natural and civilized. Tompkins shows how Graham used this simple rhetorical comparison—natural man and civilized society—to give the South Pacific a "key role to play in the United States' self-imagining" in the nineteenth century.[24]

During the Civil War, the American doctor James Salisbury treated Union soldiers with a diet of scraped beef pulp (later named the Salisbury steak). Salisbury justified his meat cure by explaining that long-lived Native

Americans and other peoples living in their "native, wild state" are "free from most of our fatal diseases," referring primarily to devastation wrought by cholera, typhoid, and tuberculosis in the squalid Union camps. Natural man only got sick "when he comes in contact with our much lauded civilization—a civilization full of 'shirking responsibility,' of sin and of the causes of disease."[25] To Salisbury, these sins of civilization must have been all too vivid: twice as many soldiers died of disease than were killed in combat in the carnage of the Civil War.

John Harvey Kellogg also celebrated Pacific Islanders and the vegetarian diets of "primitive man." In *The Natural Diet of Man* (1923), Kellogg railed against unnatural, modern "palate-tickling and tongue-blistering sauces" of "gustatory enjoyment," insisting that plain, fleshless diets produced strong, upright people. He included Friendly Islanders (now Tongans) and Ladrone Islanders in his list of mostly vegetarian peoples who "exhibit extraordinary strength and endurance. . . . Modern man is a very old-fashioned animal, but he is trying to live in an altogether new and unbiologic manner," Kellogg concluded.[26]

In the 1930s, the American dentist Weston Price traveled the world documenting the relationship of primitive diet to tooth decay, later publishing the influential 1939 *Nutrition and Physical Degeneration* and, four years later, *Health Lessons from Primitive Living*. Sometimes called the "Darwin of Nutrition," Weston Price's work continues to inspire diet books that venerate diets of "primitive" peoples. In 1999, the Weston A. Price Foundation was established to restore "nutrient-dense foods to the human diet" by honoring the "wise and nurturing traditions of our ancestors."[27] The Price Foundation models itself on attention to the "diets of healthy, nonindustrialized peoples [that] contain no refined or denatured foods" and has unified many of the earlier precontact and primitive diets.[28] Similarly, the Ancestral Health Society officially organized in 2009 to offer a "new direction in physiology that respects our evolutionary heritage as human beings."[29] Broadly, Ancestral Health Society, the Price Foundation, and the precontact diet movement overlap with the scholarly or pseudo-scholarly fields of nutritional epigenetics, evolutionary gastronomy, and Darwinian dietetics.

Precontact diet books along with organizations like these offer insight into how non-Native people practice primitive diets. Medical research also informs these popular diets as well as obesity and diabetes treatment. *Diabetes Care, American Journal of Clinical Nutrition*, and reports published by the World Health Organization (WHO) uncover the consequences of these stories. This chapter pays particular attention to the career of Paul Zimmet, the foundation director of the International Diabetes Institute, whose research on Aboriginal Australians and Pacific populations has been published in *Diabetes Care* and other leading journals since the late 1970s. News outlets in the United Kingdom, mainland United States, Hawaii, and Australia provide geographic diversity. Interviews and correspondence with Terry Shintani complement a study of published sources.

First published in 1997, Dr. Terry Shintani's *The HawaiiDiet*™ is the best example of a mainstream Pacific Islands weight loss diet.[30] The book set off a wave of publicity in presses in Hawaii and the mainland, developing out of the earlier success of his Wai'anae Diet Program, a "strict, traditional Hawaiian diet" composed of "foods eaten in Hawaii before the onset of Western influence" to induce weight loss in twenty-one Native Hawaiian participants.[31] The president of the Hawaii Health Foundation and a caring, if bullish, medical leader, Shintani offers the standard timeline for Hawaiian precontact diets: positioning his diet before Captain Cook's arrival in 1778 because, as he mistakenly believes, "we know that prior to that, there was no outside influence."[32] "Before they were subject to Western influences," he explains, "the Hawaiian population flourished, nurtured to health in an environment of pure water, a warm climate and lush vegetation." Native Hawaiians were "naturally trim and athletic," he explains, because they "lived in harmony with the universe." In my interview, Shintani said that if you lived before Cook, you might "pick fruit from the trees in the mountains; if you had a friend who was a fisherman, he might come up and once in a while you might have fish. It would all be in with the rhythm of nature."[33] In *The HawaiiDiet*, Shintani writes that successful dieters "intuitively understand nature and the universe as our ancestors did. . . . Our bodies, minds, and spirits will begin to resonate with nature."[34]

Native voices are also integral to any Pacific-centered understanding of diet advice. Anthropological research has shown the majority of Samoan food activists and entrepreneurs also view the past as healthier, linking freshness to health in "a nostalgic past before the influences of globalization."[35] Activist Claire Ku'uleilani Hughes, writing in a 2012 issue of *Ka Wai Ola*, describes her ancestors as "lean, muscular, and athletic," but "we have become soft, heavy and sickly."[36] Tonga's Prime Minister Lord Tu'ivakano similarly advocated: "We have to go back to the old ways, just eating good food—taros, kumaras, yams."[37] Interviewed by the Centers for Disease Control and Prevention in 2008, activist Dofi Faasou argued for "going back" three times in as many minutes, insisting that Islanders "go back to the way our ancestors used to eat: fish, taro, at its natural form . . . if we go back to our lifestyles which our ancestors had lived . . . if we just go back to the diet of our ancestors."[38]

If the caveman diet was a fantasy of prehistory, the Pacific Islands are a fantasy of precolonial life founded on medical fact. Since the late 1970s, measured rates of obesity and associated diabetes and heart disease there have dramatically outpaced global rates. The so-called Paradise Paradox or Hawaiian Paradox has been widely recognized since the 1990s. While Hawaii touts its reputation as "the Health State," Native Hawaiians suffer from unprecedented rates of diabetes, obesity, and other conditions classi-fied as diseases of civilization.[39] The Hawaii State Department of Health in 2011 reported obesity rates topping 40 percent for Native Hawaiians.[40] By contrast, statewide obesity rates are estimated at 21.9 percent.[41] Across the Pacific Islands more broadly, a *Pacific Health Dialog* review paper reports rates as high as 50 percent for Western Samoans and 77 percent for Naurans. The United Nations Development Programme summarizes the situation in no uncertain terms: "The islanders are raising the most obese generation of humans in history."[42] Even more chilling, authorities treat Native Hawaiians as a vanishing race, speculating along with one article on cardiometabolic syndrome that no full-blood Hawaiians will live to see the year 2045.[43]

The narratives of Pacific Islands diet advice are morally tricky. They speak to nineteenth-century debates about the biology of racial difference, polygenic theories of human origins, and discourses of noble savagery and extinction. They often revive ideas considered defunct and racist. They do so in the service of people who are suffering. The colonial literary and an-thropological legacies embedded in precontact rhetoric might be a small price to pay for real-life returns: of lives saved, of pain relieved, of health restored. But hope should never be a hall pass. Given the thorny politi-cal, moral, and racial issues attendant to traditional diet and indigeneity, the historical undertow of this rhetoric cannot go unnoticed. By viewing medical research and diet advice specifically through a literary lens, this chapter analyzes the intellectual debts of contemporary Pacific Islands diet advice to Western literary traditions and nineteenth-century theories of racial difference.

Pacific Islands diet advice reproduces many themes of colonial literature: it eternalizes a timeless past, it homogenizes great diversity, it localizes
people to a fixed place, and, most broadly, it constructs the Islands as paradise, peopled by indulgent innocents, isolated from the larger world and the
advances of time. Pacific diet books invent tradition by essentializing the
Native *body* as a receptacle of historical authenticity. The "thrifty gene" hypothesis, especially, uses the diseased Native body as evidence that the sudden introduction of modernity overwhelmed the naturally slow processes
of evolution on the Pacific Islands. By arguing diabetes and obesity are diseases of civilization best fixed by a return to a mythic traditional past, these
narratives invent traditions by suggesting certain people are less compatible
with civilization.

Obesity is a tricky addition to the litany of diseases introduced by Western forces. Whooping cough, smallpox, measles, and influenza decimated
the population of the Pacific Islands. When Captain Cook came ashore in
Hawaii in 1778, some models of population growth suggest that between
800,000 and 1,000,000 Native Hawaiians populated the island.[44] In 1900,
fewer than 50,000 Native Hawaiians remained. Today, some 350,000 Native
Hawaiians or Pacific Islanders live on the islands and many more live in the
continental United States.[45] This outdated vision of fatal impact persists:
obesity and diabetes are weakening the population and the purity of the
race is at stake. Blaming poor lifestyle choices and laziness complicates fatal
impact theory, perhaps contributing to the recent resurgence of the "vic-
tim-driven view of the Pacific past," as Barrie Macdonald puts it.[46] And so
too many diet experts tell Islanders to revert to the old ways because modern diets aren't for them.

Even diet books without any ostensible connection to the Pacific draw
upon Pacific themes. A chapter titled "A Traditional Pacific Islander Diet"
in the 2012 bestselling *Perfect Health Diet*, for example, admires the "traditional diets of the Pacific Islands, where inhabitants were noted for their ex-
ceptional health and beauty." The authors recommend breadfruit, coconut,
fish, squid, seaweed, algae, pork, fowl, and shellfish as healthful elements of
the "traditional diet of the native Hawaiian."[47] Nearly all plans begin with the
moment before "the arrival of modern civilization."[48] Other popular diets
use the Pacific Islands as a parable about the dangers of processed foods
and rapid westernization. Like Margaret Mead's lessons of sexual permissiveness, these epidemics are used as mirrors—or, as diabetes researchers

put it, a "natural experiment"—for Westerners to meditate on their poor eating habits.[49] The 2011 *21-Day Weight Loss Kickstart*, for example, praises the "de-spammed" traditional diet while decrying the "fatty food tsunami" of the "Western import [of] hamburgers, chicken nuggets, cheese pizza, or fried chicken" that swept diabetes and obesity onto the Marshall Islands.[50] Other diets glean broad themes from the epidemics: the 2004 *Tropical Diet* or the 2005 *The Coconut Diet* promise dieters will become "healthy, trim, energetic, and alive" if they follow the "*nutritionally exotic*" diet that once kept "tropical islanders trim and healthy."[51]

It can be difficult to clearly separate diet from diet books. Diet in the Pacific Islands is a hugely complex issue, understood best by analyzing racial histories, colonial legacies, sovereignty struggles, and economic inequalities. Cuisine, tastes, and the many different Islander philosophies of food should also be accounted for, perhaps by paying particular attention to the notion of embodied memory and inequality so successfully recognized in recent work like Julie McMullin's *The Healthy Ancestor: Embodied Inequality and the Revitalization of Native Hawai'ian Health*. Scores of Islander doctors are tackling the disease burden of noncommunicable conditions like obesity, diabetes, and some cancers. Food First and other food justice and sovereignty groups organize conferences, lead tours, and teach traditional cooking courses. Poets, artists, and musicians raise awareness about obesity and disease.[52] All this good work deserves credit and respect.

Diet books have little to add to these discussions. Diet books regularly confuse and misidentify Marshallese, Filipinos, Native Hawaiians, Naurans, Tongans, Samoans, and even South Asians (in one embarrassing instance) in the hodge-podge mix of poi and piña coladas that make up the Pacific Islands in the American cultural imaginary. They often grossly misrepresent Islander history, politics, or even basic geography. Yet geographic or historical accuracy is not usually a standard held to diet books and the mistakes are telling. Popular diet advice does flatten and disrespect the diversity of the Pacific Islands, but these inaccuracies reveal debts to the literary and intellectual legacies that similarly misunderstand the Pacific.

Diet books ignore the serious issues of sovereignty, race, and inequality because they are dreams, myths, the hopeful stuff of stories. It would be easy to dismiss diet books and other myths because they are, in fact, fictions, but fictions told as fact are often more telling than fact. Hope is so often a poor disguise for despair; an imagined future reveals much about the harsh realities of the present. By examining the dreams of the Pacific Islands diet book without condemning them for ignorance or insensitivity, we can better understand not what is true but what ideas about diabetes and obesity on the Pacific Islands are *tendered* as truthful. After all, what other genre not only promises "revolution" and "hope to the diseased" but also offers precise instructions to "achieve perfect health and maintain it through a long life"?[53] Diet books are best read not to call out ignorance but rather to understand myths. Only by fully and carefully studying these myths—for their meanings, their historical undertow, their utopian promises—can we see them truly as the stories we tell ourselves about ourselves and, perhaps, a story for which we can write a better plot.

Several historiographical traditions also provide perspective. Diabetes is cast as an aggressive pathogenic Western force invading and upsetting the fragile ecologies of the Pacific Islands and Pacific Islanders, drawing from discourses of noble savagery. Called "one of the most persistent themes in Pacific historiography," the notion that "western culture had devastating cultural and biological consequences for islanders" veers toward neo-Darwinist ideas of fatal impact or extinction theories.[54] James Clifford's "timelines" of non-Western others and his refutation of "rootedness" help situate the precontact diet in related movements, particularly nineteenth-century discourses of civilization. The diets also add the decline of health to the four narratives of decline—political, moral, environmental, and intellectual—that Oliver Bennett has argued characterize the counter-Enlightenment tradition of twentieth-century Western cultural pessimism.[55] When read alongside Sander Gilman's history of obesity, Bennett's insights suggest that these diets belong to larger narrative structures of historical decline.[56]

Such scholarly and historical perspectives help make sense of the language of timelessness, of paradise lost, of the essentially Pacific body, of the bounded local, and of "eating in place" saturating the precontact diet movement. In just a few sentences, Gary Paul Nabhan, professor and locavore leader, distills centuries of colonial literature in his 2004 book on gene-food interaction and cultural diversity. Observing the Pacific Ocean "in a garden of healing plants," Nabhan hears "the deep bass sound of a conch shell [that] blew us back into a more ancient time, or perhaps, into a *timelessness*."[57] After filling his plate with taro corms and fish, he remarks, "When

I turned around and looked back into the dining pavilion, I saw a sea of jubilant Native Hawaiian faces. They were pleased—if not jubilant—to once
again be *eating in place, eating with their ancestors, and eating what was fit for
their genes and their cultural identity*."[58]

There is a fine line between "eating in place" and knowing one's place. A
moral tightrope separates well-meaning people from helping those who are
suffering and unintentionally reinscribing the very colonial tropes they seek
to upend.

FATAL IMPACT AND THE "LESSON FROM THE PACIFIC"

Obesity and other noncommunicable diseases are often considered recent
(or at least mid-twentieth-century) additions to the list of the "ghastly
scourges" introduced by Western invasion. Before Price, very rarely did
non-Native observers recognize how diet contributed to poor health. Instead, epidemics of communicable disease such as typhoid, influenza,
measles, and leprosy were held liable for Native Hawaiian and Tahitian
population loss.[59] Dental photographs (Figure 3.1) served as evidence that
poor nutrition corroded teeth and caused decay. Generalizing across the
Pacific, Price observes:

> In the past some of the natives have had splendid physiques, fine counte-
> nances, and some of the women have had beautiful features. They are now a
> sick and dying primitive group. They have largely ceased to depend on the sea
> for food. Tooth decay was rampant. . . . The individuals living entirely on na-
> tive foods were few. Some early navigators were so highly impressed with the
> beauty and health of these people that they reported the Marquesas Islands as
> the Garden of Eden.[60]

Price's vision of the precontact Pacific is rich with allusions laid by Paul
Gauguin, John La Farge, Herman Melville, Henry Adams, and other late
nineteenth- and early twentieth-century Western artists and writers. With
what Renato Rosaldo aptly terms "imperialist nostalgia," these artists use
a "pose of 'innocent yearning' both to capture people's imaginations and
to conceal its complicity with often brutal domination."[61] Inspired by
Melville's 1846 novel based on the Marquesas Islands, John La Farge's 1895

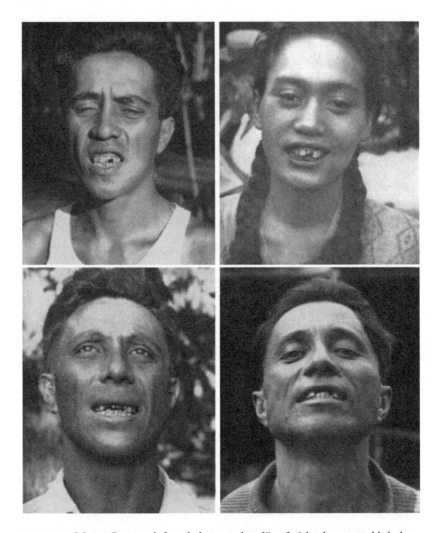

FIGURE 3.1. Weston Price took dental photographs of Pacific Islanders to establish the relationship between tooth decay and a "civilized" diet, first publishing these images in dentistry trade journals in 1935 and later reprinting them in his popular 1939 book, *Nutrition and Physical Degeneration*. These photographs depict tooth decay in "typical modernized Tahitians."

Fayaway Sails Her Boat, Samoa (Figure 3.2), is most powerful for what it suggests but does not say outright. Fayaway subdues nature with nature, revealing her beauty in the very moment she uses her robe to catch the wind and power her canoe. La Farge points toward Rosaldo's "brutal domination" by

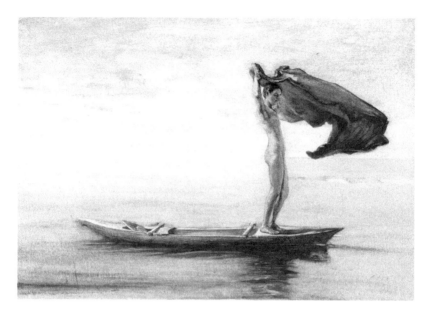

FIGURE 3.2. John La Farge's 1895 *Fayaway Sails Her Boat, Samoa* depicts a passage in Herman Melville's 1846 novel, *Typee: A Peep at Polynesian Life.* Melville describes a beautiful young woman who disrobes and uses her loincloth to sail her canoe. Melville called her a pretty little mast and La Farge's watercolor of the scene is considered one his greatest artistic achievements. Private collection.

pacifying it and Fayaway tells a harmless tale of nature subdued. Using her own loincloth as a sail, she recasts the mechanics of colonial power—sailing, ships, the conquest of nature—as a peaceful, feminine embodiment of uncorrupted sensuality.

If La Farge prematurely mourned a myth of Fayaway, Western narratives today mourn a corrupted, now-obese Fayaway whose tragedy portends doom for the human race. No one better summarizes this than health guru Paul Bragg, reflecting on Price's research and writing: "The effects of Western civilization's diet of death on other races is more rapid and therefore more apparent than what we are doing to ourselves. But the white man is eating his way out of existence."[62] Media and medical research still regularly report on the "lesson from the Pacific," claiming that isolated islands act as a "natural experiment" for testing the cause and consequence of Western diet and disease.[63] "The remote and idyllic atolls of the Pacific Ocean" act as one microcosm for global trends, Zimmet observes in a 2000 article

subtitled "Can the Doomsday Scenario Be Averted?"[64] Many of these studies approach the Pacific as a parable, an experiment, a lesson to be learned
and a fate to be avoided.

These narratives replicate many of Alan Moorehead's views on "fatal impact," a term coined in his 1966 study of late eighteenth- and early nineteenth-
century exploration of the South Pacific. Fatal impact theory, following
closely with ideas of the "dying savage," presents a victim-oriented view of Pacific colonization blaming European explorers and subsequent colonists for
ruining the Pacific Islands and Pacific Islanders. As Doug Munro and Brij V.
Lal observe, Moorehead was only naming a "familiar tradition, articulating
long-held views about the dire effects of European wickedness on an innocent island world."[65] And health has long been a metric by which to measure
Pacific Island devastation: scholars regularly cite eighteenth-century evidence to show how the "ghastly scourges" of tuberculosis, mumps, typhoid,
and so on visibly ravaged the Islands, causing the "precipitous decline of
this formerly robust population."[66]

Even government reports rely on suspect first-account narratives to condemn "civilization" for the current epidemics. A 2003 World Health Organization report recounts, "Upon European contact, Pacific people were
described as strong, muscular and mostly in good health."[67] The report, pre-
pared for a major conference, Food Safety and Quality in the Pacific, cites:
"Descriptions given by the early European explorers provide evidence. The
French explorer Louis de Bougainville recorded that the Tahitians were almost godlike and lived in an environment overflowing with natural abundance: 'I never saw men better made' and 'I thought I was transported into
the garden of Eden.'" After reviewing nutritional profiles of over a dozen Pacific Islands, the authors suggest that "reverting back to traditional lifestyles
and foods" would help the inhabitants regain that original health.[68]

Epidemics of noncommunicable disease have flipped Moorehead's language on its side: the obese are blamed in ways that people infected with
influenza or whooping cough would never be. Even though the blame
might be passed from invader to victim, the narrative structures remain
stable: a precontact "innocent island world" meekly crumbling, without
choice or agency, under the deadly weight of European disease. Caught
in the binary of blameworthy and blameless, this structure both elides the
politics that accompanied the disease and the agency of the Islanders that
resisted its spread. The blame baton is passed from one party to the other,

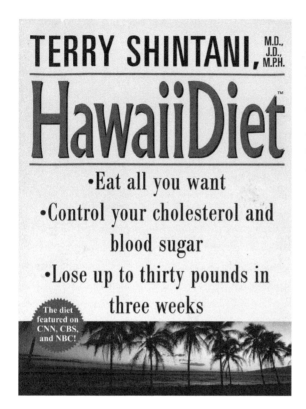

FIGURE 3.3. Terry Shintani's 1997 low-fat Hawaii Diet grew from his 1994 study called the Wai'anae Diet Program that prescribed a strictly traditional Hawaiian diet to induce weight loss in twenty-one Native Hawaiians.

ping-ponging liability and generating a lot of bickering but little action or understanding.

EMBODIED UTOPIA AND *THE HAWAIIDIET*

Shintani's 1997 diet book offers the most concise, popular, and representative account of the precontact diet story (Figure 3.3). The Hawaii Diet plan is simple: a low-fat, high-fiber, high-carbohydrate program roughly described as based on a "premodern" Hawaiian cuisine and crops native to Hawaii. Cooking methods rely on steaming, baking, broiling, or roasting, described earlier as "a manner that approximates ancient styles of cooking."[69] Recipes are mainly grouped according to course. Soups, salads, beans, rice, potatoes, and desserts all merit their own section. "Traditional Hawaiian Foods," however, is grouped on its own and includes recipes for "'*Ono* Taro Tops," "*Lomi* Tomato," "Vegetable Laulau," and nine other dishes. Other recipes include Portuguese Bean Soup, Tofu Mayonnaise, Quick Mexican Pizza, and Ratatouille. In fact, Shintani categorizes only twelve of the more than 150 recipes in *The HawaiiDiet* as traditionally Hawaiian. Granted, fusion cuisine reflects the rich diversity of Hawaiian food cultures.[70] Historical accuracy is also by no means expected of a weight loss diet but, by setting aside "Traditional Hawaiian Foods" into its own section, Shintani shows he isn't mistakenly categorizing Parmesan cheese and guacamole as part of a traditional Hawaiian diet. Rather, he uses those twelve recipes to add authenticity to a conventional and somewhat grim low-fat diet of tofu and bean soup.

Shintani bypasses rational nutritional calculations and privileges the body and its natural instincts: satiety is the main measurement of the Hawaii Diet. Most diet programs like Weight Watchers calculate nutritional components or otherwise weigh, measure, or quantify the foods of the daily diet. However, Shintani says, "I didn't want to say eat so many grams of this, grams of fat" or "oh don't eat meat the size of the deck of cards" because this type of thinking "is so foreign" to Native Hawaiians. "This wouldn't resonate with the Native Hawaiians—most people wouldn't know what a gram is," he continues, so Shintani relied on the body's natural processes of satiety and hunger to construct the Shintani mass index, for which he offered the acronym SMI.[71] SMI measures volume against energy to calculate how useful certain foods are to the weight loss endeavor, bypassing the reckonings of the dieter and relying instead on the body's instinctive feelings of fullness.

In the published version, Shintani claims that the Hawaii Diet does not rely on "rigorous willpower" or the "calorie counting or portion-size restriction" of most weight loss diets. Rather, the Hawaii Diet "utilizes your natural enjoyment of eating," allowing the dieter to skip the rational calculations of typical weight loss programs and simply relish "healthy, delicious foods that satisfy in every way."[72] This logic maintains the "innocence" of the body by foregrounding "natural" appetites in evaluating the success of the diet plan.

Shintani also believes that the healthfulness of Hawaiian cuisine lies not only in the nutritional profile of taro and yams (or Portuguese bean soup), but also in the spirit of aloha, the pure landscape of precontact Hawaii, and the "ancient wisdom" of Native Hawaiian ancestors. *The*

Tropical Diet similarly claims, "A complete state of tropical wellness was about everything the islands offered, not just the diet alone."[73] Similarly, Nabhan insists that his diet will "renew the vital connections between your body and the land that are essential to restoring health at all levels."[74] Likewise, as a "whole-person program," the Hawaii Diet includes "an understanding of universal principles embodied in traditional Hawaiian beliefs."[75] A return to traditional Hawaiian health, then, entails a mythic process of time travel—by body, in time, over land—to a place akin to what Rob Wilson calls the "primordial purity, holistic happiness, and unchanging authenticity" used to describe "some kind of bounded, well-knit Pacific community."[76]

The Hawaiian landscape bound up in Shintani's imagination of the Hawaiian body draws from a rich American intellectual tradition, inspired by Emerson, that configures the landscape as an antimodern cure for civilization and its diseases. "Ancient Hawaiians were very spiritual," Shintani claims, so they understood "that food, land, water and health were inseparable."[77] Much of precontact diet advice suggests that the most pernicious diseases of civilization come from a bodily alienation from nature. Their regimens prescribe an intimacy with nature as the solution to obesity, but situate this curative landscape in the past. Tinged with poetic loss, this landscape is described as unmediated, bountiful, and natural. It overflows with fresh fruits and vegetables, ripe for the picking, and so supplies an antimodern antidote to the rampant overprocessing and commodification of food.

Nature is imagined as everything the contemporary Pacific Islands and Islanders are not or have lost.[78] That sense of loss imbues descriptions of traditional diet—for example, that the "diet was based on fish caught from the sea, for example, or mangoes and other fruits picked from the forests." An Edenic vision of leisure erases the demanding and sophisticated Native farm labor and agricultural system that predate Western contact, all clearly evident in studies of Native irrigation, dryland planting, wet-farming zones, and other farming methods. The Edenic abundance and ease is set in sharp relief to current ways of life. For example, one report found that Naurans "confess" that they binge four times a day, "adding, 'after finishing a meal and lying in front of the TV for an hour, you soon get hungry again.'"[79] Journalists add that the "palm trees, ivory beaches, and a languid lifestyle" are tourist dreams. "In Nauru, a popular snack is a whole fried chicken, washed down with a bucket-sized beaker of Coke."[80]

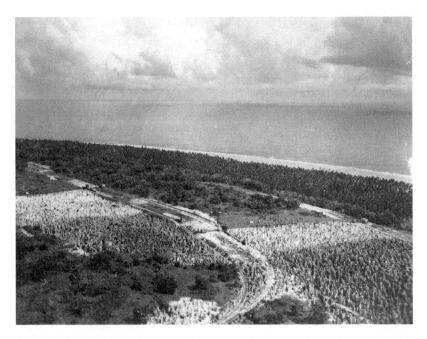

FIGURE 3.4. 1942 photograph of phosphate mines in Nauru after the British Phosphate Commission left behind a wasteland of barren coral pinnacles. Courtesy State Library of Queensland.

However, this poetic loss is historically accurate for many of the Pacific Islands. Colonialism did deplete or ravage many of the Islands and foreclose traditional sources of nutrition—fishing, for instance, or land-intensive crops. As one Hawaiian activist puts it, "In talking about health, you must talk about food, so you must talk lo'i (gardens)—and so you've got to talk golf courses, and so you've got to talk foreign investments."[81] The gardens *do* depend on the golf courses, especially for tiny islands like the eight-square-mile nation of Nauru.

Nauru has become a cautionary tale about the costs of civilization in public health circles and many diets use Nauru's collapse to link the twinned forces of environmental devastation and obesity/diabetes. Called "the fattest place on Earth," the tiny island nation was literally carried off by British and Australian interests when they strip-mined it for valuable phosphate deposits (Figure 3.4). After independence in 1968, the Nauran government wrung the land for all it was worth, creating nearly total resource exhaustion and now over 80 percent of the total land area has been strip-mined for the valuable chemical.

Nauru's sudden postcolonial wealth from phosphorous mining rocketed the world's smallest nation to the top of two world rankings: for a few years in the 1970s, per capita income for Naurans was the highest in the world and Naurans also suffered from some of the world's highest rates of obesity and diabetes. Over 65 percent of Naurans were obese and nearly half diabetic. Amid widespread media coverage, diet leaders nearly always referenced the massive environmental wreckage phosphate mining left on the tiny, now-ugly island, prescribing a diet that remembers the pre-phosphate island environment and way of life. In the wake of the 2015 refugee crisis, Nauru expanded its contract with Australia to house detention facilities. Hundreds of emaciated asylum-seekers have staged hunger strikes to protest brutal conditions, sewing their lips shut with twine and refusing food for days. For some, the contrast between Native Naurans and thin refugees illustrates the tragedy of the crisis.[82]

Much more is at stake than pounds lost or diseases cured: the diets respond to the historical forces of colonialism and development, of loss and devastation, of the actual past as well as the remembered one. Rhetorically, the diet enlists Islanders in a unifying utopian vision of shared health, showing how one healthy person improves the health of the world. "You will be invited to participate in a great movement to restore the good health of all the Hawaiian people," the *Wai'anae Book of Hawaiian Health* promises.[83] Shintani told me his ultimate goal was "to create a social movement" with the Wai'anae Diet, which was later printed as a small pink book. Mahatma Gandhi wrote "the green book," Shintani said, and "this is my answer to that: I wrote the pink book."[84]

Shintani's diet is a utopian vision that imagines a past and promises a future by pivoting on the most immediate aspect of the present: the body and its many daily needs. Utopia is a slippery concept, but Lyman Tower Sargent offers the best description. It is "social dreaming" that expresses in practice, literature, and social theory the desire for a better world—and, by "showing everyday life transformed," utopias depict a better way of *being* and *living* in that better world.[85] Diet advice promises to transform the most banal, bodily kinds of being—eating, exercising, drinking water or tea or kava—in the larger project of health, broadly defined. To borrow Shintani's words, his diet will inaugurate "world health and world peace," if only dieters "begin with the health of the individuals who make up the world." A dieter's success will be one step "to heal ourselves and our world."[86] The project of the perfectible body becomes bound up into visions like Shintani's that enlist the individual to make a better world.

INVENTED TRADITIONS: THE BODY
AS TEMPORAL CONTINUITY

Diets like Shintani's are not merely utopian dreams of poi-filled paradises but active, fluid inventions of tradition. These traditions rely—not on lore or law—but on the Native body to construct a vision of history already laid and derived in the U.S. imagination of the Pacific Islands. The body is key to understanding the invention of tradition as corporeal, as alive, as constantly being-made in the endless interpretation of history. These diets uncover the *practices* of historical memory and tradition by casting the Native Hawaiian body as a receptacle of historical authenticity.

Richard Handler and Jocelyn Linnekin have argued that "tradition" is an interpretive process, treated "less as artifactual assemblage than a process of thought—an ongoing interpretation of the past."[87] Conceptually, the notion of tradition rests on the continuity of past with the present. As Eric Hobsbawm and Terence Ranger have shown, tradition is always an invention of the present—useful fictions that help shape some vision of the future by recasting it in terms of the past.[88] In Ranger's view, the invention of Native traditions has long served the imperialist project. In a Foucauldian sense, these measures of "authenticity" are internalized in the body of the indigenous subject, reinforced through prescriptions as banal as what and how to eat.[89]

Tradition is never a benign rumination on the past but a tool—or a weapon—used to steer the future. Tradition selects parts of the past, silences others, and makes history anew. Put another way, the stories of *there and then* say more about the *here and now*: "Tradition is a model of the past," Handler and Linnekin note, and this model "is inseparable from the interpretation of the tradition in the present."[90] By reframing traditional diet not as a historical fact but as a collection of invented traditions, we can move beyond asking whether these diets "work" but instead ask what they *mean*—what this particular collection of taro and prayer invented as traditional tells us about the culture that invented it. How do these diets contribute to discourse about modernity, progress, and the "diseases of civilization"?

According to Shintani and other advocates, Native Hawaiian bodies conserve nutritional instinct and retain their connection to ancestral heritage. Shintani told me, "Hawaiians have this common experience, and common knowledge about what happened. They still have the memories of their grandparents and their parents" and the diet "reaches inside people to what's already there."[91] Kauila Clark, an activist for Native Hawaiian health, articulates a similar model of the body and temporal continuity, arguing "the indigenous foods are the foods that have ensured that you are here. You are a survivor in your family—your people made it for thousands of years on these foods, and you, right now are the continuing link."[92] Even if paradise has long been lost, this model of the Native body uses the body to link past to present to future, so providing the temporal continuity necessary for invented tradition.

The Native Hawaiian body has long been entwined with political projects of sovereignty that rely on memories of the past to make claims for rights in the present. Blood quantum requirements also link body, land, and belonging in contemporary Hawaiian identity politics.[93] When land dispossession posed a political threat in the 1990s, anthropologist Cari Costanzo Kapur shows how the Native Hawaiian nationalist movement emphasized "natural, historical, and cosmological 'rootedness'"—a celebration of indigenous taro farmers, for instance—or how the "genealogical connections to the taro plant, and Hawaiian lands, occupy collective memory."[94] At other times, the nationalist movement remembered mobility, particularly the "history of Polynesian seafaring expertise . . . in the 1970's and 80's" when politically advantageous.[95] Like this arm of indigenous blood- or land-based activism, Pacific Islands diet advice treats "ancient" bloodlines or ancestral bodies as continuous with the past and so sharing a special relationship to Native lands in the present.

As Gayatri Spivak puts it, "strategic essentialism" can be politically useful to nationalist activism, but it also limits the range of identity and expression.[96] Essentialism is particularly risky in the precontact diet because, unlike blood- or land-based activism, the *diseased* body could be misconstrued as essentially Native Hawaiian or Pacific Islander. By framing diabetes and obesity as "diseases of civilization" and markers of indigeneity, the diets implicate diabetes and obesity as evidence that certain bodies are less compatible with civilization. Perhaps due to a growing awareness of the "interactive cosmopolitanism" of so-called localized Natives, these diets and diet advice redirect the "long temporal continuity" of tradition away from the Islander culture and into the body of the Islander, reframing the "diseases of civilization" as embodied, visible products of the threats civilization poses to natural indigenousness.

Alongside medical ecology and Darwinian gastronomy, precontact diets claim that certain people are "optimally adapted" to certain environments. If they depart from traditional ways, disease will ensue. Shintani has argued that since the "inherent healthiness of the land" nurtured Native Hawaiians, food is still the Native Hawaiian's "connection to the land—the minerals, the chemicals, the land and water and so forth.""When you eat in harmony with the land," Shintani says, then true health envelopes body, mind, and spirit.[97] Implicit in his argument is a twofold localization of food and people: it is this kind of "localization" that scholars Geoffrey White and Ty P. Kāwika Tengan have noted as a disciplinary fault with many early studies of Pacific Island life. White and Tengan observe, "One reason Pacific Islanders have been reluctant to embrace the paradigm of anthropology is precisely their interest, historically, in resisting consignment to bounded local spaces, to a depiction of 'traditions' as fixed, limited, and set in opposition to modernity."[98] Diet advice insists Islanders are adapted to both a place and a time. Through the invented traditions of a "Native" diet, the diets commit the body of a people to a body of land and a mythic past.

Just as fieldwork as a methodology is rooted in specific geographies, Pacific diet advice emphasizes rootedness and tends to fix people and place, cementing the seemingly natural relationship between land and people. This logic essentializes the connection between Native people and Native lands but ventures one step further: essentializing the *body* as a vessel of historical memory, authenticity, and continuity. James Clifford has pointed out that "assumptions of rootedness and local continuity, notions of authenticity" have denied many indigenous groups "complex agency in an interactive, ongoing colonial history."[99] Even when Pacific Islanders no longer live on "ancestral lands," diet advice recommends Island crops and cuisine. Even though she now lives in Utah, Dofi Fassou supports "going back" to the cuisine of her native Tonga/Samoa. This is not to support what one scholar has called the "pernicious notion that indigenous people who do not live in [their] homeland become less native," but rather demonstrates how this diet discourse literalizes and essentializes the connection between body and land.[100]

This recalls a fundamental intellectual clash between two theories of race, debating whether the human race's common heritage trumps superficial differences in diet and lifestyle or if these differences should determine ideal ways of life. Native diets offer a history of human origins based on the essential difference between people—in this case, Natives and Westerners, or those ostensibly better adapted to a Western diet and modern life. Both the Paleolithic and Eden diets follow a different model, clearly arguing for a single origin of the human race and prescribing the same ancestral or "original" diet for all human beings. No matter religion, race, or generation, the advice is the same: eat like the caveman or eat like Adam and Eve, our common ancestors.

These competing origin stories fall neatly into the major intellectual debate about race in the nineteenth century—between monogenism and polygenism. Much more accepted today, monogenism posits a single origin of humanity and both the Paleo and Eden diets follow a monogenic model of common shared ancestry. Polygenism contends that different human races are of different origins, something suggested by the precontact diet view that certain people are optimally adapted to certain diets and ways of life. The intellectual history of polygenic or monogenic debates about human origins is long, contentious, and, at first glance, seems like an ugly relic of outdated intellectualizing. However, the intellectual lineage is clear in contemporary diets. Like most polygenic diets, the precontact diet offers a modified version of the theory of biological recapitulation. Rather than group human beings from different lineages of the same age, these polygenic origin diets group humans according to their particular moment of historical emergence. In other words, certain human beings have "newer" ancestry than others. Accordingly, these diets modify the biological theory of recapitulation by cutting phylogeny off short; put another way, something interrupted the chronological recitation of the successive evolution of the human species, retarding or slowing down evolutionary progress. However, instead of mapping an individual's development onto the evolution of the human race, polygenic diets segment all contemporary human beings into categories—racial or otherwise—and position each category at one rung on the long ladder of evolutionary development.

Precontact diets are not alone in suggesting polygenic origins. In fact, a slew of recent "blood type" diet books use polygenism as their central claim. Few of these diet books claim human *races* require different diets, but they all use some inherent body-category to determine difference, whether blood type, body shape, taste sensitivities, weight storage patterns, or racial descent. These books argue for the indelibility of history in the human body, yet rather than claiming shared origins, they group, characterize, or otherwise lump human beings into different diets based on differences established by a spectrum of quantitative metrics.

Most polygenic diets resist explicit racial categories in prescribing appropriate weight loss plans—for example, the popular "body typing" diets such as the 2001 *Different Bodies, Different Diets* or the 2005 *The Body Shape Solution to Weight Loss and Wellness*.[101] Body type or body shape diets follow an older form of "somatotyping," or the process best remembered as psychologist William Herbert Sheldon's 1940s categories of endomorph (round, pudgy), ectomorph (tall, thin), and mesomorph (triangular, muscular). Sheldon's taxonomies were rife with "racist and eugenic subtexts" about racial, physical, and intellectual superiority. Even in his own time, other psychologists disowned Sheldon for his "fascist pseudo-science," but those categories live on in body type diets.[102] In fact, his legacy is thanked in a half-dozen diet book introductions and explicitly invoked in diets ranging from the 2004 *Look Great Naked* to the 2012 *12-Day Body Shaping Miracle*.

Hopefully, Sheldon's racist views got lost in the shuffle from his 1940s psychological treatise to *Look Great Naked*. But other diets such as blood typing programs take race-based polygenism as their most essential premise. Though based on seemingly objective blood typing, a close reading of the first popular "type" diet, Peter D'Adamo's 1996 *Eat Right 4 Your Type* diet, reveals a complex typology of race, place, time, evolution, and diet. Like Shintani, D'Adamo uses inherent difference to trace out a creation story. D'Adamo argues that "blood types are as fundamental as creation itself" and "follow an unbroken trail from the earliest moment of human creation." In literal terms, bloodlines "are the signature of our ancient ancestors on the indestructible parchment of history."[103]

D'Adamo's diet breaks down the human race into four different types: Type O, Type A, Type B, and Type AB. D'Adamo's timeline divides people into degrees of ancientness: the "o" in Type O stands for "old" and represents hunter-gatherers, Type A is for "agrarian" types who emerged in the

New Stone Age, Type B is for "balance," and, finally Type AB is the modern type developed from the "intermingling of Type A Caucasians and Type B Mongolians."[104] Type O bodies, for example, require high-protein diets and intense aerobic exercise while Type A dieters fare better on vegetables, tofu, and light exercise. Recipes provided for Lamb and Asparagus Stew and Quinoa Apple Sauce Cakes, for example, are older dishes designed solely for Type Os.

By laying out this chronology, D'Adamo's diet positions certain types of people in both time and place. "Each of the basic races has its own homeland" but "as human races migrated and interbred," new types developed and people lost sight of the "inherent, instinctual messages of our biologic natures." Blood Type O, or "old," started in Africa, Type A in the Middle East and Asia, and Type B originated in the Himalayan highlands. D'Adamo philosophizes that modern Type AB is harder to locate and could serve as "the perfect metaphor for modern life: complex and unsettled." The book ranked in the bottom 10 percent for "nutritional adequacy" among popular diet books, but despite the lack of scientific or medical corroboration, it was a blockbuster.[105] D'Adamo reported in a 2016 revised edition that *Eat Right 4 Your Type* has been translated into sixty-five languages and sold over seven million copies.[106]

A slew of recent DNA or gene diets claim that our ancestral lines are complex enough to warrant entirely unique nutritional requirements. Like other primitive diets, DNA diets are modeled after ancestral health but temper the possible racial implications of the claim by explaining that every person's unique ancestry warrants a "bespoke" diet. The 2016 *DNA Restart: Unlock Your Personal Genetic Code to Eat for Your Genes, Lose Weight, and Reverse Aging* claims "our modern life is simply out of touch with our DNA." Referring to the dieter's distinct ancestry, the author Sharon Moalem laments, "We've turned our backs on the wisdom contained within our three-billion-letter genetic code that our forbearers spent thousands of generations carefully annotating and preparing for us." Even though ancestral wisdom is "locked away deep within our bodies," Moalem's plan will "unlock your DNA's hidden dietary rules that have been crafted specifically and only for you."[107]

DNA Restart is polygenism at its finest: instead of Shintani's Native versus Westerner types or D'Adamo's four types of human being, Moalem claims there are six million types of human being and each type has evolved over a different period of time. And since "eating for someone else's genes can be deadly," every human being needs personal and specific diet recommendations, helpfully supplied by *DNA Restart*.[108] If the Hawaiian diets link people to a place first and to a time (the past) second, then *Eat Right 4 Your Type* links people to a time first and to a place second. The DNA diets dodge the question of what group of humans came first by explaining that every human sits on a different rung of the evolutionary ladder and every diet is unique to every rung.

The *HawaiiDiet, Eat Right 4 Your Type,* and *DNA Restart* belong to a long tradition of categorizing people by place, race, and time. Historically, place and local foods were paramount to many nineteenth-century thinkers' empirical bases for polygenism. By the late nineteenth century, polygenic thinkers used Darwin's theories to support their ideas of separate origins. Herbert Spencer and other theorists applied ideas of natural selection to theorize for the coexisting stages of racial development in humans, suggesting that different races could have descended from apes at different times. Spencer and others argued that "savages" like Australian Tasmanians or American Indians represented a previous stage of human evolution. Spencer and his colleagues contended that since human beings belonged to different species or different stages of the evolution of species, diet was only influential to a point. Diet could shade the complexion or enfeeble the figure, not transform races from one species into another or leapfrog a people into a more advanced evolutionary stage.

By the same token, even eighteenth-century theorist Samuel Stanhope Smith balanced his fundamentally monogenic view with his belief that climate and diet changed physical characteristics. His 1787 book is "now considered the most important work on race in its generation," and, in it, Smith proposed the now-conventional view that climate caused racial differences such as skin color and height.[109] Still, Smith believed that less advanced peoples were more susceptible to climate and diet, arguing in an 1810 edition, "Climate exerts its full influence, and produces its most deteriorating effects in a savage state of society."[110] Food, in particular, determined the cultivation of society and the beauty of a people. "Every change in diet," Smith claims, "and every variety in the manner of cooking and preparing it for use, is accompanied with some alteration in the system."[111] Diet advice today replicates that sentiment, suggesting that the most primitive peoples are the hardest hit by changes in diet.

TIME AND TIMELESSNESS: THE ANTHROPOLOGICAL LEGACY OF ETERNALIZING

In the narrative imaginary of the precontact diets, the local places of the Pacific Islands are imbricated with notions of mythic or long-lost time. Or, as one article in the *Journal of the National Cancer Institute* phrased it, "For centuries, time had seemed to stand still in the territory of Papua New Guinea," depicting a place outside time and people unaccustomed to change, like ants in amber.[112] As scholars including Johannes Fabian, James Clifford, and Chandra Talpade Mohanty have noted, anthropological writing tends to situate others on the "before" point of the timeline of human progress. After Fabian, Clifford observes the "pervasive tendency to prefigure others in a temporally distinct, but locatable, space (earlier) within an assumed progress of Western history."[113] Like the distinction between country and city, Clifford shows how other opposites align: "civilized and primitive, 'West and non-West,' future and past."[114] The notion of the primitive encapsulates time and place: non-West and the past are bound together in some vague receding horizon.

The concept of the past in the non-West is also less chronological and more timeless than similar notions of Western progression. Renato Rosaldo calls this process the "eternalizing" of a timeless and somehow more homogenous Native culture.[115] One of Zimmet's early findings is responsible for the near ubiquity of this eternalizing tendency in Pacific diet advice. In the late 1970s, Zimmet concluded that the sudden introduction of modernity overwhelmed the slower processes of evolution on the Pacific Islands. He writes:

> While populations of the Western world went through enormous social and technological revolutions in the last two centuries, the Pacific Islanders and their social, cultural, and economic patterns had remained untouched. . . . In the space of a few years, the Pacific Islanders were parachuted into the 20th century. While Western societies had a gradual introduction to its new technology and scientific progress over several centuries, the process was telescoped into a period of less than 30 years in most Pacific countries.[116]

Zimmet's conclusion has largely been upheld in subsequent scholarship published in *Diabetes Care* and widely cited in the popular press, like one

Foreign Policy paper that argues, "It's not piña coladas. Evolution has been overwhelmed by Western lifestyles."[117]

Zimmet's narrative isolates and marginalizes the concurrent advances on the Islands, wedding place and time in ways that eternalize and homogenize Pacific Island cultures. Not only do these narratives of decline imply that a faster rate of change characterized history in the Western world but they also regard obesity and diabetes as evidence of the success of the Western invasion. As Sander Gilman notes, this concept of globalization and original health "postulates a model not so much of change but of invasion . . . a modern version of 'degeneracy theory,' with the new assumption that the ills of the world are to be traced directly back to the developed world."[118]

Researchers often blame civilization itself—not just Spam and soda—for interrupting this timeless paradise with modern ills. Georg Forster, who accompanied Captain Cook on his trip to Tahiti in 1773, found that, in the natural abundance of Tahiti, "gluttony was impossible, as only in a society of inadequacy did the passion for food arise." "Fat men were impossible in Tahiti," a seemingly perfect natural society, he added, far from the stresses of competition linked to high rates of diabetes and obesity.[119] Today, the foreign imports of consumerism and stress have reversed that situation. In the same influential article investigating the "medical effects of social progress," Zimmet writes that "an easy-going Pacific Islander may find the change to a desk job or the responsibilities of a senior civil service post quite stressful in relation to his previous traditional lifestyle."[120] Echoing Zimmet's sentiment nearly twenty-five years later, Michael Curtis writes in the *Journal of Development and Social Transformation*, "The significant changes connected with the transition to a cash economy have also brought great stress to the people," which he counts as a risk factor for obesity and diabetes.[121] Obesity is also blamed on consumerism, a statement made by a 1987 article reprinted in *Pacific Health Dialog* in 2003 describing how "consumerism is rife in the Pacific Islands, with its avaricious fingers increasingly extending out to and touching even the most isolated rural areas and outer islands." The media revolution, with its "uncontrolled introduction of television" might be the "most pervasive and powerful promoter of consumerism and nutrition-related ill health in the Pacific Islands."[122] Another 2014 Islands-centered publication remembers that, before Westerners, Islanders "were perfectly adapted to their environment, lived in harmony with their ecosystems and free of the compulsions of unbridled consumption of consumer goods."[123]

In all these narratives, diabetes and obesity are framed as the tragic costs paid by Islanders for civilization. Disease is bound into other supposedly foreign imports, ignoring all the technological accomplishments, sophisticated systems of economic exchange, and advanced agricultural methods that predate Captain Cook. Primitive diet advice assumes an agential Western force that intruded on a timeless, untroubled paradise and, as we will see, retains traditions set by colonial literature and described as "twentieth-century lotus-eater fiction." Taken from Greek mythology, the term "lotus-eater" depicts people drugged by the apathy-inducing effects of the delectable, irresistible lotus plant. Paul Lyons describes how lotus-eater fiction "softens and eroticizes Oceania," referencing examples of the "sensuous storytelling mode" that celebrated the islands as cocoons of warmth, peace, and security.[124] As a 1931 Eugene O'Neill character described the lands—full of "warm earth in the moonlight—the trade wind in the coco palms—the surf on the reef . . . the natives dancing naked and innocent—without knowledge of sin!"[125]

The nutritionally liberal attitude of Islanders follows in traditions portraying sexual permissiveness, most familiarly in Margaret Mead's *Coming of Age in Samoa*. The two are tangled in culturally relativistic reports aghast that Pacific Islanders could find fat appealing: "In fact, islanders even today admire plump women, seen everywhere here in billowing big T-shirts over long skirts, with plastic flip-flops on their feet," one typical report accounts.[126] Curtis calls unhealthy beauty ideals a "challenge to health policy implementation," summarizing the situation in three words: "*big is beautiful*."[127] Just as Odysseus describes the lotus as "so delicious that those who ate of it left off caring about home" or thinking of the future, similar language depicts the obese Islander basking in pure sensuality and unthinkingly succumbing to the siren song of dangerous foods.

Fatty meats—mutton flaps, Spam, corned beef, and turkey tails—have generated much discussion about Islander appetites for meats called inedible or disgusting to Western palates since World War II.[128] Called "stigmatized foods" regarded as "too fatty to be eaten by the (mostly) white people who produce and purvey them," anthropologists have described the "politically charged" commerce as "a First to Third World trade that brings the epitome of fatty meat to those with the epitome of fatty bodies."[129] In 2007, Samoa's Prime Minister Tuilaepa Sailele Malielegaoi banned imports of turkey tails—the oily gland colloquially known as turkey butts—to reduce epidemic rates of obesity in his country. The ban was later lifted upon Samoa's 2013 accession into the World Trade Organization.[130] A typical report in the *Global Mail* describes the "greasy, bitter and rancid" fat-and-gristle of turkey tails as unpalatable to "westerners, and even most Americans." Considering these tastes as an "addiction to fatty meat," the reporter concludes that, with the lift of the 2007 ban, that "Samoans will again be able to indulge their morbid appetite for the very worst kind of junk food."[131]

In tone and tenor, the language describing these "morbid appetites" and "frighteningly sumptuous" Island feasts recalls other Western fears about cannibalism, another wanton Island appetite. One writer postulated "that former cannibals of Oceania now feasted on Spam because Spam came the nearest to approximating the porky taste of human flesh."[132] Though it's in jest (corned beef has a "corpsy flavor"), the humor reveals the persistence of cannibalistic discourses about Island diets. Scholarship has long been squeamish about the appetite in studies of primary reports of cannibalism. Non-Native histories, however, are rich with descriptions of the delectability of "people-meat" to Pacific Islanders. British artist Augustus Earle called this "unjustifiable cannibalism" in his account, since appetite alone—not revenge or passion—prompted the "infernal feasts."[133] In his well-regarded 1948 *Anatomy of Paradise*, J. C. Furnas argues that the Fijian "cannibalized for gastronomic reasons. He *liked* man-meat."[134] By 1951, Douglas Oliver hedges about cannibalistic pleasures in *The Pacific Islands*, arguing that "such ingestion" was mostly "not done for nourishment but for one social purpose or another." "Nevertheless," he prevaricates, "there are many credible accounts of Islanders having killed and eaten for gustatory pleasure."[135]

Equally prurient, almost salacious language characterizes many Western discussions of other taboo meats. "It's fatty, it's juicy, it's tasty, it's moist," one radio respondent described turkey tails.[136] "In the U.S., the tails of turkeys are deemed inedible" but are thought tasty by many Pacific peoples, one public health report said gently.[137] Less mildly, a 2007 *National Post* article writes that, "where once Pacific peoples ate reef fish and yams, they now gorge themselves on corned beef and 'turkey tails'—cheap, highly fatty pieces of skin."[138] Still more direct, a 2006 *Guardian* report claims that "Tongans are eating themselves to death" with the "frighteningly sumptuous" feasts of sucking pig and other fatty tidbits.[139]

Following the tradition of cannibalistic discourses, Islanders' "morbid appetites" dictate their diet, even when taught that these appetites are disgusting or deadly. The liberal explanation for the epidemics still focuses on the Native appetite but shifts the blame from insatiable appetites to the so-called thrifty gene, or the genetic disposition to gain weight first postulated in 1962 by population geneticist James Neel. The hypothesis has wide traction today. A *National Post* article acknowledges that "Tongans, for instance, are believed to be predisposed to weight gain and are poorly equipped to deal with processed food."[140] The *Guardian* nods to the thrifty gene but blames the paradisiacal environment: "It is an uphill struggle to make dramatic lifestyle changes when you already live in paradise," the reporter observes, especially because Tongans "aren't aspirational in the worldly sense" and "many don't seem keen to do much at all, apart from cooking."[141]

As with many genetic explanations for disease, the thrifty gene hypothesis can sometimes veer dangerously toward biological determinism and social Darwinism. According to one public health scholar, this "thrifty gene" hypothesis "has led to a kind of fatalism and therapeutic nihilism which is quickly transferred to patients and their relatives."[142] In either account, Islanders just "can't help it" and Western foods are portrayed like the lotus—narcotic and addictive, seducing Pacific Island appetites with the fatty delights of tinned meats.

THE PROMISE OF PARADISE

In *Typee*, Herman Melville asked a question of the "once smiling and populous Hawaiian islands." Were the fruits of civilization worth it for the "now diseased, starving, and dying natives"?[143] More than a hundred years after Melville, similar questions are still being asked. One headline speculates that obese Tongans might be fat and "happy—but should they be worried?"[144] Or, as the United Nations Development Programme asks: are the people of the South Pacific "Trading Health for Wealth"?[145]

Some questions are better asked than answered. But we can always question that line of questioning—and then question the kind of world that would think to ask these questions. The intellectual links of Pacific Islands diet advice to Western literary and anthropological legacies are, at best, riddled with well-intended clumsiness—at worst, willful ignorance. The ways they are riddled are not random, however, but rhythmic. These stories of disease in the Pacific Islands are, indeed, stories too often limited to legacies laid by old literature and old anthropology and old ways of thinking. Both diet advice and these traditions lean on similar modes of narration, and both rely on the same historical referents, likely because both are products of a culture that for too long has imagined the Islands as paradise, Islanders as innocents, and disease as the sad, inevitable product of westernization.

4 ❧ DETOXIFICATION DIETS AND CONCEPTS OF A TOXIC MODERNITY

W̶EIGHT LOSS DIETS have long been left out of the histories of food politics and activism in the United States. However, a new story emerges when we include detox diets in the history of food politics. Beginning in the 1980s, detoxification or "detox" diets generated new ideas and concepts that later became critical to political discussions of food, health, and obesity in the United States. In particular, detox diets expanded the drug and alcohol addiction framework to include food addiction and invented the notion of the "toxic food environment." Maybe books like Michael Pollan's 2006 *The Omnivore's Dilemma* or Marion Nestle's 2007 *What to Eat* are not new and different food manifestos but simply two texts in the longer history of the continued politicization of the diet book.

The concept of toxicity also sidesteps some thorny political questions about personal responsibility and the role of government in the rise of the obesity epidemic in the United States. As Abigail Saguy notes in her study of obesity, Americans have used three primary "blame frames" to explain the epidemic. Conservatives often favor the personal responsibility blame frame that holds obese people directly liable for their poor lifestyle choices. Liberals usually prefer the sociocultural blame frame, turning instead to patterns of poverty, urban planning, agricultural subsidies, and the food and beverage industry to explain skyrocketing obesity rates.[1] The third, less contentious blame frame, rationalizes the epidemic with biological or genetic arguments, a concept better known as "endogenous" obesity caused by a slow metabolism or other innate biological mechanisms.[2]

The politics of obesity in the United States often pit the first and second blame frame against each other. Conservatives fight for consumer freedom and personal choice while liberals advocate for government regulation and policy change. Very rarely is there a middle ground between these opposing points of view. Yet detox diets combine both perspectives with some unlikely sleight of hand by invoking the concept of toxic food addiction—the idea that Americans are physically addicted to unnatural, toxic foods and live in an unhealthy environment that disposes them to those food addictions. Simply put, the detox argument goes like this: Americans are unhealthy because they make bad choices, but Americans make bad choices because they are addicted to toxic junk foods and live in an unhealthy environment. The blame might rightly lie in American culture and politics, but the onus is still on the individual to regulate what he or she eats.

Detoxification diets also helped introduce the metaphor of toxicity into public discussions about food, addiction, and obesity in the United States. Beginning in the 1990s, obesity prevention researchers and alternative food activists used the "toxic food environment" to explain food addiction and rising obesity rates. This argument—like detox more generally—uses the concept of food addiction and toxic environments to mediate between conservative arguments for personal responsibility and liberal beliefs in government intervention. Toxicity is the middle man in the relationship between environment and citizen—the go-between that begins with the environment and ends in the body of the obese American. Very few diets pinpoint actual toxic substances like mercury in tuna fish or preservatives in processed foods. Instead, toxic foods or a toxic society are easy scapegoats in the blame game of food politics in the United States because "toxins" are nearly always general, vague metaphors for all that is wrong with American culture, politics, and people.

Unlike more traditional weight loss diets, detoxification diets are not specifically for the overweight or those looking to lose weight. In the detoxification framework, *everyone* is exposed to some unhealthy level of toxic load. One early detox diet asserted that detox is for "every individual that breathes air, eats food, and drinks water."[3] Some detox books even claim that fetuses can be poisoned as toxins travel through the permeable placenta.[4] Breastfed babies are equally vulnerable. Detoxification diets also promise much more than weight loss—freedom from disease, newfound purity, unexpected energy. One detoxer told me that, though she hoped to lose weight, she also believed that she "would look shinier" after her week-long lemonade fast. "I would look like I was beaming with light and I would be happy—I would feel happy," she said.[5]

In practical terms, detox diets have changed little since the late 1980s. Most often, these diets are low-calorie, short-term fasts of fruit or vegetable juices like the infamous Master Cleanse Detox, a diet of lemon juice, maple syrup, and cayenne pepper. Some diets supplement detoxifying foods with practices such as ionic footbaths, colonic irrigation, and enemas. Others recommend mental or spiritual detoxification like visualization or deep breathing. Still others provide herbal or homeopathic cures for disease. But all subscribe to the same fundamental notion that, by diet, detoxers can purge the harmful, septic substances out of their toxic bodies and lives.

In cultural terms, detox diets reveal new ways that Americans have conceptualized the effects of modern living and the postindustrial environment on their health. Like hippie food movements before them, detox diets have considered individual health as inextricable from the larger systems of global capital, industrial development, and social structures. Detox broadens the one-directional argument of environmentalism, showing that, just as humans pollute the environment, that polluted environment retaliates and hurts human health. As a metaphor, toxins mark the porousness of the boundary between environment and body, suggesting the ways in which Americans have understood their relationship to the changing physical world. Detox diets are also particularly critical of American culture and politics because the diets blame the total toxic environment at large—nutritional, physical, cultural, social—for poor health. An analysis of detox diets, then, is by proxy an analysis of how Americans understood themselves and their culture at the turn of the twentieth century. In particular, detox diets give observers of American culture fresh windows into new concepts of addiction, changing perspectives on environmentalism, and more focused insights into the origins of the alternative food movement.

In the last ten years, detox diets have exploded. Detoxification diets, products, and services are among the most popular diet programs in the United States. Detox diets have appeared on *The New York Times* bestseller list every year since 2008. There are detox spas, clubs, magazines, and gyms, as well as countless detox products and devices ranging from organic colonics and electrified footbaths to juices and vitamins. A 2009 estimate by the International Spa Association showed that "almost all of the roughly 15,000 day and destination spas nationwide offer some kind of detoxifying treatment" that can range from a $15 pedicure to a $4,500 weekend retreat."[6] There are specialized detox plans for armpits, toenails, and the scalp. Celebrity "detoxers" include Beyoncé Knowles, Oprah Winfrey, and Salma Hayek.[7]

All this in spite of the firm denunciation from nearly all reputable doctors. Researchers have called such diets a sham, a con, a waste of time and money, "tantamount to fraud," and "nonsense for the gullible."[8] A recent president of the American Dietetic Association said, "Detox diets prey on the vulnerability of dieters."[9] Some detox diet doctors are charlatans, posing with fake medical credentials and guaranteeing miracles. Some are respected medical leaders with verified credentials. Yet both regularly promise incredible things: the cure for diabetes and heart disease, fast and painless weight loss, and renewed vitality. Many are like Roni DeLuz, PhD in "natural health" and a certified hypnotherapist and colonic therapist. DeLuz's 2007 book promises dieters they can lose a pound a day following her instructions for Asparagus Detox Juice and Creamy Nutmeg Broccoli Soup. DeLuz charges $695 a day for her detox retreat in Martha's Vineyard. She sells cancer treatment kits through her website.[10]

Some are like Mark Hyman, the bestselling author of *The 10-Day Detox Diet*. Hyman has served as a consultant to the surgeon general, presented at the World Economic Forum, and has been featured in both Katie Couric's 2014 film *Fed Up* and in the Clinton Global Initiative. Hyman doesn't outright promise miracles, but he does offer examples of dieters losing eleven pounds in three days, curing their diabetes, and overcoming food cravings with the "restorative magic of biology." Science and magic mix as Hyman touts the "magic in the 10-Day Detox Diet" even as he insists his diet is "not a magic cure or a gimmicky weight loss scheme."[11] Despite Hyman's quackish language and outlandish claims, his diet has resounded with mainstream and respectable audiences. None other than Bill Clinton blurbed Hyman's bestseller.

Detox has come to mean so much in just four decades: a cure for cocaine addiction, a yuppie fad, a celebrity ruse, a hippie cult, and, now, a presidential weight loss program. How has the movement come to mean so much for so many? What has detox offered American culture and how has it changed? This chapter draws from a survey of more than a hundred detox diet books.

FOOD ADDICTS IN A TOXIC ENVIRONMENT

Insight can be found in one of the earliest detox diet books, *Detox* by Merla Zellerbach and coauthor Phyllis Saifer. *Detox* offers an origin story for the forty-year detox tradition, shedding light on the diet's two most important contributions: insights into changing concepts of environmentalism and addiction and reflections on the odd combining of idiosyncratic ideas by practitioners of detox. Zellerbach wrote *Detox* in 1984 to warn Americans of "widespread toxic contamination," which she considered "a major public-health problem of the twentieth century." The diet itself was complicated: foods were divided into families and then each family followed a specific rotation every four days. All these foods could only be cooked with spring or filtered water in specific materials: stainless steel, glass, porcelain, and cast iron were permissible, but aluminum, nonstick, and plastic cookware were prohibited due to possible contamination of the food. Coffee, vinegars, alcohol, sugars, and processed and premixed foods were also verboten.

For example, on the first and third days of the diet, detoxers could eat from the citrus, gourd, crustacean, or palm food groups. On the second and fourth day, the olive, myrtle, mollusk, and grape families were permitted. A sample menu outlined the first-day diet to include oatmeal, roast lamb without skin, and cucumber sticks. Day two would rotate food families to include tuna with alfalfa, skinless chicken with grapes, and cabbage salad with raisins. After rotating the food families for two days, detoxers would be expected to feel "lighter, bouncier, and more alert within forty-eight hours."[12]

Of the two hundred pages of text, only ten pages are devoted exclusively to this diet. The remaining pages describe what toxins are, how they affect the human body, and general advice on topics ranging from alcoholism to water quality. Zellerbach sidelines the actual food plan by offering only four recipes for the diet: tomato-beef broth, green sauce, parsley-chicken soup, and Waldorf salad. Zellerbach directs readers to consult other cookbooks for more recipes.

Zellerbach's promotion of detox was unusual for her social station. Until her death in 2014, Zellerbach was a prominent San Francisco socialite and philanthropist with an impressive publishing record in the *San Francisco Chronicle* (Figure 4.1). She served as editor of the *Nob Hill Gazette* for more than a decade and wrote romantic fiction on the side. Zellerbach was more Berkeley than Bel Air and a far cry from the Southern California yuppie New Agers who saw detox as a shortcut to weight loss. Zellerbach's *Detox* was politically informed and she reproved industrialization and the two world wars for introducing into the environment chlorine, mustard gases, and DDT.

Zellerbach's *Detox* was an obviously environmentalist text. The book opens with these two sentences: "It is now a fact that harmful substances are everywhere: in the air we breathe, the water we drink, the fresh vegetables we eat, and the clothes we wear. The environment, once so familiar and trustworthy, is becoming a stranger as toxic chemicals permeate our atmosphere, lakes, oceans, and soil."[13] Later, Zellerbach recounts a condensed history of environmental pollution, explaining how nineteenth-century forensic medicine invented toxicology, 1920s industrial food processing contaminated food with rodent debris and dirt, and World War II "launched an era of synthetic chemicals."

Zellerbach was smart about her environmentalism. She took all the fury of Rachel Carson and tempered it with the easy, familiar language of a diet book. Carson called toxins the "elixirs of death" in her landmark 1962 *Silent Spring*. By contrast, Zellerbach calls toxins "universally injurious." Carson diagrammed organic compounds of hydrogen, carbon, and chlorine to explain how chemists had "produced a battery of poisons of truly extraordinary power."[14] Zellerbach gives practical advice to avoid household toxins,

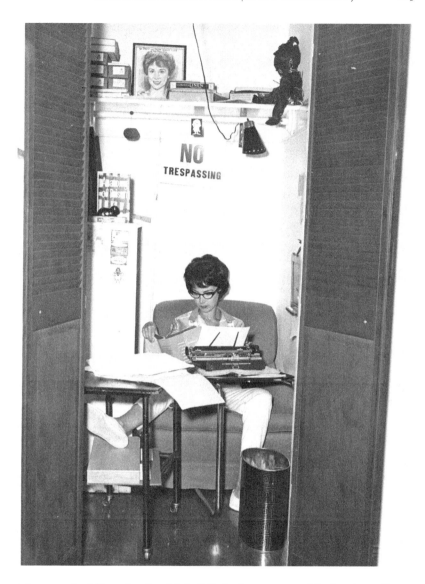

FIGURE 4.1. Socialite and author Merla Zellerbach wrote one of the first detox diets in 1984. *Detox* combined environmentalist concerns with new concepts of food addiction. Pictured here in her home office in San Francisco. Courtesy Gary Zellerbach.

assuring readers that, for many toxins, "damage is usually temporary and heals when use is discontinued."[15] Carson and Zellerbach shared an environmentalist stance, but Zellerbach softened Carson's alarmism by giving her readers an easy, relatable, step-by-step process to think about and act against toxins.

Heralding the detox movement, Zellerbach did not stress policy change or even personal consumer activism, but instead turned inward to hearth and health. She instructs readers to close their house windows on smoggy days, roll up car windows in cities, use unscented cosmetics, and, of course, keep a keen eye on their diet. Though Zellerbach did include the contact information of environmental action groups (Friends of the Earth, for example, and the U.S. Environmental Protection Agency) in an appendix, the primary focus of her book is personal. "We can live clean lives in a polluted world," she predicts, and, for Zellerbach, detoxification is "a valid and effective answer to widespread toxic contamination."[16]

Environmentalists could easily criticize this approach as a retreat—making the political so personal that the politics drain out entirely. True, Zellerbach advises her readers to eke out a clean, detoxified corner of that world for themselves and their families. Yet she refuses to accept environmental damage as irrevocable and promises that the future could look more like the past, before toxins seeped into American food and water and air and land. In a way, Zellerbach uses selfishness as a springboard, promoting a diet to rally self-concerned readers not simply to improve their own lives but to save the world. This sentiment is clearest in her last chapter:

> On an individual level, we have learned how to detoxify our bodies and keep them that way. There is no doubt that we can live clean lives in a polluted world. We cannot, however, dissociate our fate from the fate of the earth. What we have learned about freeing our bodies from harmful substances must also apply to cleaning up the world. . . . By the year 2000, we should all be breathing cleaner air, eating unprocessed and uncontaminated foods, and drinking water that is fit to drink.[17]

Zellerbach's *Detox* was also among the first few texts to broaden the addiction framework to include everyday foods like wheat, corn, eggs, or beef. Since the 1970s, food activists had likened sugar and caffeine to addictive drugs. John Yudkin's 1972 *Pure, White, and Deadly* (recently reprinted with the subtitle *How Sugar Is Killing Us and What We Can Do to Stop It*) suggested a not-so-subtle comparison to cocaine. William Dufty's 1975 bestseller *Sugar Blues* claimed that refined sugar was a lethal, addictive substance that acted much like a dangerous narcotic. Subtlety was not Dufty's strong suit. "Heroin is nothing but a chemical," Dufty writes, adding that "sugar is nothing but a chemical" refined into "strange white crystals."[18] Something of a pop culture sensation, *Sugar Blues* was promoted by none other than Gloria Swanson, Dufty's wife at the time.[19]

"Food addiction" was first coined in a 1956 paper by allergist Theron Randolph, but his definition of addiction more closely resembles today's conceptualization of an allergy—an uncoordinated, sometimes unnoticed reaction to a specific food. Not widely known until the 1970s, Randolph's work matured into an alarming "addiction pyramid" in 1980 in which all food was a gateway drug. Randolph conflates addiction with the basic biological need to eat: food addiction was a necessary dependence that, according to his pyramid, quickly drove addicts from proteins and sugars to glues, solvents, and opiates like heroin.[20] Randolph's peculiar brand of "clinical ecology" was one of many disciplines to adopt the ecological model; environmental historian John Opie explains that "nonscientists turned to ecology as a model for philosophy, humanities and social sciences."[21] Like detox, clinical ecology also used the insidious dangers of modern food to reflect the "hazards of modern civilization" but within the framework of diet and allergy, not weight or diet-related disease.[22]

It wasn't until Food Addicts Anonymous was established in Florida in 1987 that obesity and food addiction became firmly linked. The organization grew most rapidly in the late 1990s.[23] Unlike Zellerbach, these organizations often classify certain foods as particularly addictive: highly palatable combinations of salt, sugar, and fat in junk foods and sweets. Over the last twenty-five years, food addiction has broadened and inspired "eating addiction," a disorder in which an addict can be victimized by any food, regardless of its composition. True, broccoli is unlikely to trigger a binge but eating addiction shifts the focus away from the food itself and toward the eater's relationship to food. If addicts have disordered relationships with food in general, they could ostensibly be equally addicted to broccoli or Big Macs.

While *Sugar Blues* and Randolph's older addiction model likely influenced Zellerbach, she was among the first diet book authors to include wheat and meat alongside cocaine and alcohol as addictive substances. Both concepts of addictive foods and eating addictions were unfamiliar when Zellerbach wrote *Detox* in 1984.[24] Zellerbach's work anticipated both concepts in her claim that *any* food could be addictive. In her chapter titled

"Addiction and Withdrawal," Zellerbach profiles "Camilla P." Without knowing it, Camilla P. had become "hooked on wheat." Zellerbach explains that Camilla P. was suffering from withdrawal symptoms (grouchiness and anger) after she ate lunches of fruit and cottage cheese. Dinner rolls, crackers, and cookies all gave Camilla P. her fix and, without wheat, Camilla P. began to withdraw from her addiction. When a doctor advised her to quit bakery products, Camilla P. endured jittery nerves, stomach cramps, and urinary frequency but, after three days, she no longer "felt the urge to attack the cookie jar."[25]

Sugar, caffeine, and alcohol were easy targets, but, Zellerbach warns, "some foods, such as milk and wheat, contain opioids—morphine-like substances—and are therefore more likely to be addictants." "Do you often find it impossible to resist eating a certain food?" she asks. Or "Do you ever feel desperate—that you would go anywhere or pay any price for that food?"[26] If yes, Zellerbach cautions, you may have a food addiction.

FOOD ADDICTS AND DIET JUNKIES

It is easy to imagine why food addiction entered popular discourse about food in America during this time. Drug use and obesity were both huge public health scares in the 1970s and 80s. Just as President Nixon declared his "war on drugs" in 1971, obesity rates were growing rapidly.[27] In many ways, cocaine and obesity were twin health scares—they were widespread, terrifying, and preyed particularly on young people and middle-of-the-road Americans. The discourse of drug addiction firmly connected body and a toxic environment, especially as the language of urban blight and urban decay made its way into popular parlance. "Drug dens" and "crack houses" soon followed in the early 1980s. Activists and artists also condemned toxicity by linking drug use, urban decay, and pollution. In 1982, street artist John Fekner spray-painted "TOXIC JUNKIE" on a "well-used drug den" in a drug-riddled part of New York City, tagging both the urban environment and drug addiction as equally toxic. Recently reflecting back on his 1982 spray-painting (Figure 4.2), he argued that "manifestations of toxicity was [sic] rampant not only by poisoning of the planet, but by those who chose a complete disregard for one's existence with the recreational use of hard drugs."[28]

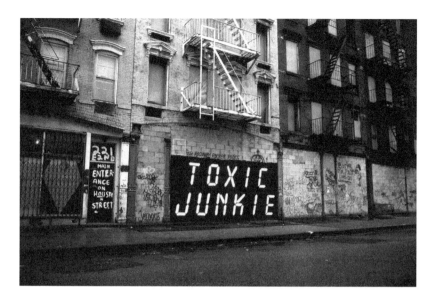

FIGURE 4.2. Environmental artist John Fekner spray-painted the words "toxic junkie" on a New York City drug den in 1982. In physically tagging the landscape, Fekner categorized drug addiction, urban blight, and the larger environmental destruction as broadly toxic. Courtesy John Fekner.

Both modern foods and contemporary drugs were linked to the high-paced speed of American life, suggesting that a dangerously fast world could at once produce cocaine addicts and sugar junkies. Gloria Swanson drew the comparison in 1977, saying, "It's considered chic for adults to dabble with cocaine, whereas [for] adolescents it's candy."[29]

As the decade wore on, Zellerbach's claims began to look conservative as diet authors started to label people diet junkies, food addicts, or sugar junkies and used the language of fix, high, withdrawal, and crash to describe these food addictions. *Sugar Blues* was one of many diet books to borrow addiction terminology. Also popular were portmanteaus that combined a specific food with "-holic," as in sugarholic or chocoholic.[30] A 1988 article in *Mademoiselle* subtitled "Are You a Diet Addict?" expanded the connection once more, warning readers about addiction to dieting itself. "Diet junkies" are characterized as women who, despite running into health problems, continued to diet and use diet helpers such as laxatives or diet pills. Blurring into growing concern about anorexia and other eating disorders in the United

States, the *Mademoiselle* article cautions readers about the downward spiral of compulsive dieting. Yet the article is breezy, reassuring readers that compulsive dieting is not a disease and definitely not an eating disorder. "You don't have to be anorectic or bulimic to be a diet addict, although diet addiction can lead to both anorexia and bulimia," the article clarifies.[31]

Actress and comedian Renée Taylor published an autobiographical account of her weight struggles in *My Life on a Diet: Confessions of a Hollywood Diet Junkie* in 1986. With a light touch, Taylor reminisced about her bizarre dieting history that included gems like the Rockefeller Spaghetti Diet, the Royal Queen Mother's Diet, and Joan Crawford's Kelp. Taylor referred to her Hunza diet secrets, a subject critical to the veneration of the "primitive diet" in the United States. Taylor alternately said she was a food addict, a diet addict, addicted to food, and a diet junkie.[32] The same year, a 1986 book diet titled *The Mollen Method* even reversed the direction of addiction, asking readers, "But how would you like to be turned on to *positive* addiction—addiction to health?"[33] Mollen called his low-fat diet the "minimum addictive dose for a lifetime of health." Continuing the theme of addiction, in 1990 Madonna quipped that she was a "sugar junkie" because she was deprived of love as a child.[34]

Diet pills also united the concepts of diet and addiction. As early as the 1930s, a toxic chemical called dinitrophenol caused blindness and death in would-be dieters. Though the Food, Drug, and Cosmetic Act of 1938 banned many dangerous drugs made popular by the new field of obesity research, common remedies such as Kruschen Salts were still readily available.[35] Thyroid hormone and amphetamines were popular as appetite suppressants well into the 1960s. Over 45,000 women developed lung and heart problems from the infamous fen-phen diet pill in the 1990s.[36] About six million Americans took the deadly drug until it was finally removed from the market in 1997 after a series of lawsuits.[37] Controversies like these had long put diet pills in the news, but diet pill *addiction* didn't appear on the national radar until 1987. In that campaign year, Kitty Dukakis, wife of presidential candidate Governor Michael Dukakis of Massachusetts, revealed she had earlier sought treatment for her lengthy diet pill addiction. Dukakis was first prescribed amphetamine pills in 1956, when she was only nineteen.[38] Public disclosures of diet pill addictions like Dukakis's brought national attention to these concerns of diet, addiction, and toxins (whether in drugs or food).[39]

Detox and alcoholism were even more pointedly linked in the United Kingdom. British newspapers and magazines caught on a few years later and began to profile detoxes extensively in the late 1990s, usually with an alcohol-themed twist. The Liver Detox Diet recommended seven days of unprocessed foods to help the liver survive parties and barbeques. The weeklong program featured raw beetroot, brown rice pudding, and ground psyllium hulls to beat hangovers and lose weight.[40] Another London paper profiled a detox diet as the "72-hour hangover cure."[41] January was a popular time to run detox articles, appealing both to dieters with New Year's resolutions and those who "are still feeling sluggish after all that festive overindulgence," as one *Times of India* article put it in January 1998.[42]

In the United States, diets were complicating ideas of addictiveness by questioning which came first: could food addiction actually cause drug and alcohol addiction? Perhaps sugar is the gateway drug? Elson Haas's influential 1996 *The Detox Diet* posited just that. After slamming the American sugar addiction, Haas argues that "our habitual sweet tooth progresses to addictive usage of caffeine, nicotine, alcohol, and foods such as wheat, refined foods, and milk products."[43] Others figured that it didn't matter if drugs and alcohol were causing food addiction or vice versa (Figure 4.3). Americans were toxic and addicted all around or, as one 1999 book put it, "modern diet and lifestyle habits, such as alcohol, coffee, tobacco and highly refined foods, also create a toxic soup."[44]

The medical origins of "detox" also unite concepts of addiction and toxicity, whether it be in food or drugs.[45] Medically, detoxification can be defined as the short-term process by which an addict clears out the addictive substance from his or her body. Sometimes withdrawal symptoms are managed with alternate drugs but detox more often means the natural and excruciating process by which a drug addict sobers up or an alcoholic dries out. Usually the addict is physically isolated and closely supervised in detoxification centers designed for drug and alcohol addiction treatment.

Although American public health measures have long used the quarantine cure to isolate drug and alcohol addicts, these new detox centers differed from older, more institutional inebriate asylums or drunk wards. "Detox," the abbreviation for detoxification, also started coming into common use in the 1970s. The cocaine renaissance of the 1970s glamorized drug addiction and, beginning in the 1980s, celebrities flocked to expensive

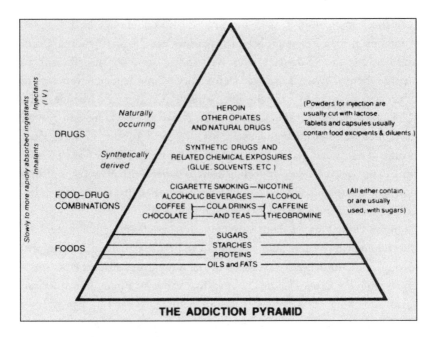

FIGURE 4.3. The allergist Theron Randolph used this addiction pyramid to show how food addiction only differs in degree of severity from addiction to heroin or other opiates. Best known today as the father of environmental medicine, Randolph first coined the term "food addiction" in 1956. Theron Randolph and Ralph Moss, *An Alternative Approach to Allergies: The New Field of Clinical Ecology Unravels the Environmental Causes of Mental and Physical Ills* (New York: Bantam Books, 1982), 21–22.

detox centers. In 1982, the $5.8-million Betty Ford Center was established near Los Angeles and attracted the likes of Elizabeth Taylor, Liza Minnelli, Johnny Cash, and Mary Tyler Moore.

From the beginning, detoxification in places like the Betty Ford Center was understood more capaciously than simple recovery from drug and alcohol addiction.[46] Detoxification might be a natural, biological process, but the shorthand "detox" suggests much more than the popularization of a medical term. Rather, detox came to suggest recovery from a *lifestyle*, a chance to purify the body from the fast-paced American culture of the 1970s and 80s. A 1985 *New Republic* article titled, punnily, "Addiction à L.A. Mode" described the process of detox not as a medical procedure designed to cure addicts of their substance abuse but, instead, as "all science can do for someone suffering the diseased life-style of the rich and famous."[47]

Certainly, the Betty Ford Center was a legitimate medical center for addictions that wrecked families and destroyed lives. The day-to-day schedule of counseling, chores, and nutritional therapy was described as grueling and harsh. The actual treatment was not particularly expensive either: fees averaged around $6,000 for a thirty-day stay, which was among the lowest in the country at the time. Insurance even covered most of these costs.[48] Yet the tragedies of actual addiction at the Betty Ford Center were often lost in the glitz and glamor of Hollywood. The tabloids crawled with speculation about which celebrities were in residence. Lavish fundraisers with towering ice sculptures and tables of sushi were attended by the likes of Julio Iglesias and Dinah Shore.[49]

Critics of detox were also critics of American culture and, not surprisingly, these detox centers and detoxification regimens were ridiculed from the start. As early as 1988, cultural critics were lambasting "detoxification" as a navel-gazing pout of yuppies in loafers and full of social pretensions. In 1989, a lifestyle columnist working for the South Florida *Sun Sentinal* included detox in his list of the "yuppification" of American English. Detox sat alongside other "semantic shenanigans" such as "palimony," "passive smoking," and "biofeedback."[50]

The best example of the use of detox to critique American culture in the late 1980s came from Legs McNeil, the fiery music journalist who gave the punk movement its name when he cofounded *Punk Magazine* in 1975. By the late 1980s, the rebellious spirit of the punk scene was on its last legs. Instead of punk, McNeil saw the "yuppie wimps who had extinguished the fires of life" becoming the "dominant social sector of society."[51] McNeil used detox as an extended metaphor by which the middle-finger attitude of a punk was replaced with the conformity and consumerism of the yuppie. For McNeil and other commentators in the late 1980s and early 90s, detox was an apt metaphor for the ways in which the politics of the 1960s or rebelliousness of the 1970s was filtered out of American culture. Without toxins, American culture was left only with the bland, narcissistic tedium of corporate culture.

This criticism aligns with political shifts at the time. Political geographer Julie Guthman studied the transition to "healthism," a term coined in 1980 that shifted the responsibility of health and disease to the individual and away from larger structural causes such as the environment or health care. Guthman argues that 1970s neoliberalism contributed to healthism because, structurally, "neoliberal governmentality shifts responsibility for care from public spheres (welfare) to personal spheres (self-help) and can depoliticize (or render futile) social struggles over resources or rights."[52] Charlotte Biltekoff expanded on the distinction between good food and the good eater, explaining that top-down nutrition advice before the 1970s quantified food and instructed Americans on the healthful diet. But with the rise of neoliberalism, "alternative dietary ideals reinforced the increasingly important social values of personal responsibility and conscious consumption."[53] But even as the blame baton was passed from the public to the private sphere, the language and criticism remained the same: pollution was killing the planet, politicians were useless, and there was something toxic about American culture itself that was poisonous to children and other living things.

If detox mansions like the Betty Ford Center and upmarket spas could cure celebrities from their "diseased life-style," then detox diets might be the poor man's version of the Betty Ford Center, catering to everyday Americans seeking respite and purification from the modern lifestyle.[54] Both detox centers and diets operated on the metaphor of addiction: cocaine and Coca-Cola could be equally addicting, many of the diets claimed, because it was the fast pace of modern life that drove Americans to speed up their minds and metabolism. As a diet—a cure for this addictive, toxic way of living—detox never stopped analyzing and criticizing modern American politics, culture, and life.

In fact, the criticism was loud and strong. Naturopaths Paul and Patricia Bragg tore into the American way of life when they promised their detoxifying diet would cure Americans diseased by a "poisoned world" in which the "big, filthy sewer in the sky" flowed down upon them.[55] One 1986 *American Health* magazine article even suggested that a detox diet could help victims of environmental disasters. "Vegetables, fruits, bran and other fibers are also helpful in ushering poisons out of the system," the authors write assuredly. With proper diet, strategic vitamin intake, and exercise, even "pollution victims may be able to detox their bodies."[56] There is something willfully naïve about recommending vitamins and whole grains in the face of actual environmental tragedies—such as the miscarriages, cancers, and birth defects of the Love Canal crisis.

A particularly pessimistic article in *Yoga Journal* described a modern world full of photochemical smog, insidious formaldehyde residues, and neurotoxic chemical fumes.[57] Even the most cautious Americans have cup-boards stocked with "foods that have been irradiated, refined, processed, sprayed, and perilously packaged in plastic." Yet in the face of "millions of pounds of chemicals" and deadly water treatment systems, the conscien-tious dieter can juice, fast, cleanse, self-purify, and meditate his way out of this deadly, toxic swamp called our "increasingly fast-paced world." *Yoga Journal* advises detoxifiers to remember a single "pearl of wisdom": that "elimination equals illumination" to guide them on the detoxification jour-ney.[58] Artist Lynda Fishbourne illustrates the advertising supplement with a yearning that belies the detox plan: the watercolor cover art depicts a woman rising up out of an industrial city, hugged by lotus flowers (Figure 4.4). Unlike other mud-dwelling plants, the lotus submerges under murky water every night, and "miraculously re-blooms in the morning without any residue on its petals." For detoxers, the immaculate lotus would symbolize purification, enlightenment, and transcendence.[59]

This kind of talk made detox diets such easy targets for punks like McNeil. Detoxers back then faced much of the same criticism that foodies do today. Without the sincerity of weight watchers or the courage of activ-ists, detoxers were left with the hypocrisy of activism-lite, criticizing Ameri-can culture with a juicer instead of a protest sign.[60] Even as it was the butt of punk rock jokes, the concept of detox was expanding to include more and more weight loss programs. As the 1990s approached, headlines like "Post-Holiday 'Detox' Starts 1991 Off Right" instructed readers about how to lose weight and cleanse toxins after the Christmas and New Year's bacchanalia. *Dr. Deal's Delicious Detox Diet Weight Loss Wellness Lifestyle* and *The Juicing Detox Diet* were published in 1992 and 1993, respectively. Both books moved away from earlier environmental prescriptions for holistic health and to-ward a stricter weight loss focus. Still they retained an antiestablishment attitude toward mainstream toxic lifestyles and industry, particularly indus-trial food processing.[61]

But by the early 2000s, the word "detox" had lost nearly all of its original drug and alcohol undertones. In 1999, one writer reflected on this shift in the *Vegetarian Times*:

> It used to be that 'detox' meant you were checking into a special facility to be
> weaned from hard-core alcohol or drug addiction. But these days, you're just
> as likely to find people using the word to describe the process of improving

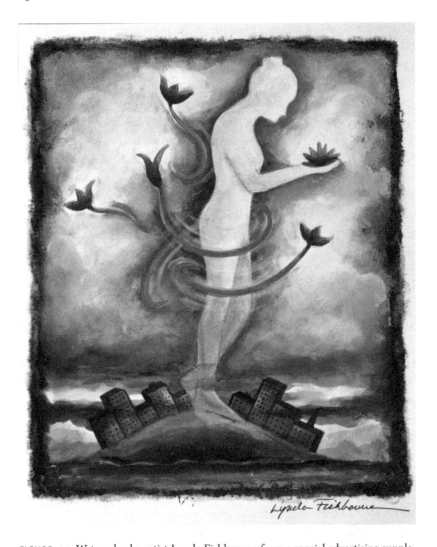

FIGURE 4.4. Watercolor by artist Lynda Fishbourne from a special advertising supplement on internal cleansing and detoxification in a 1997 issue of *Yoga Journal*. Fishbourne illustrates the promises of self-purification by painting a woman transcending an industrial city, literally rising into the clouds, wrapped by lotus flowers as symbols of purity. Courtesy Lynda Fishbourne.

their health by ridding their bodies of caffeine, tobacco, junk food and environmental pollutants. Consider detox a remedy for that chronic condition known as late-20th-century life.[62]

Firmly embedded in American concepts of health, detox now truly is a "remedy for that chronic condition known as late-20th-century life." Many detoxers treat toxins as metaphors. One interviewee described toxins as "all the preservatives and chemicals" that are "ruining the insides of my body."[63] When I pressed another interviewee for what, exactly, she was hoping to cleanse from her body after her one-week liquid fast, she said: "What I pictured in my mind was the stuff that accumulates when you've cooked bacon—the stuff that drips from fried things. That's what I imagined that was stuck in my body." She believed that, after cleansing out that thick fatty stuff, she "wouldn't feel bogged down . . . that gross, heavy, fatty feeling. I'll be freed of that, I'll be happier because my body will sense that I'm without these toxins."[64]

THE FOODIE MOVEMENT AND THE TOXIC FOOD ENVIRONMENT

Detoxification diets picked up these trends—cocaine use, food addiction, diet pill addiction, the obesity epidemic—and united them into the poignant concept of a complete toxic environment. This inescapable environment was addictive, toxic, and riddled with obesogenic foods and unhealthy ways of life. By the time the alternative food movement gathered steam in the early 2000s, detox diets were no longer the province of hippies, food faddists, homeopaths, new agers, or even people with an environmentalist bent like Merla Zellerbach. Rather, the diet began to politicize food itself and participated (and perhaps precipitated) the burgeoning alternative food movement in the first few years of the decade by introducing the concept of the toxic food environment. Unlike previous notions of addictions or individual toxicities, detox diets pioneered the concept of a complete toxic health environment particular to food and eating.

The toxic health or toxic food environment concept was first adopted in academic discussions of the obesity epidemic in the mid-1990s. Kelly Brownell, the codirector of the Yale University Center for Eating and Weight Disorders, began to use the term in 1995 in discussions of obesity-prevention drugs. Brownell argued that genetic predisposition played only a little role in determining obesity and, instead, blamed an obesogenic environment of high-fat, delicious, cleverly marketed calorific food.[65] Brownell's environmental argument complicated the old fight between endogenous or exogenous causes of obesity, the former ostensibly caused by innate biological mechanisms or conditions such as hypometabolism and the latter a product of weak willpower and poor lifestyle choices.[66] Brownell and detoxers took the environment, psychology, and biology into account, demonstrating how obesity was the unfortunate byproduct of a barely escapable way of life built on sedentary labor and highly caloric foods. Jane Brody cited Brownell's views in a prominent *New York Times* two-part column on weight loss in 1996. Brody elaborated on the toxic food environment by illustrating how Americans are "hard put to escape caloric overload when faced with mini-marts at service stations, drive-in windows at fast-food establishments, packaged fast-food meals and 'super-size' servings of high-fat, high-calorie foods."[67] For Brody and Brownell, obesogenic or "bad" foods were part and parcel of the whole toxic food environment—an environment that could be described as a poisonous American society.

Later, the toxic food environment came to incorporate American ways of work, sociality, etiquette, and family life. "We live in a toxic environment with regards to obesity," an expert noted in a *New York Times* article in 1999, explaining, "Food is very palatable, very cheap, very easy to get. Labor-saving devices are everywhere. Everybody is working at desks."[68] "We are, in short, eating ourselves to death in a strange exercise in slow-motion communal foundering," another news commentary observed in 2004.[69] If the toxic "communal foundering" was causing obesity, then detox could leverage community to cure obesity; a later detox author promised just that, claiming the "community was the cure and that most chronic illness—including obesity—was in fact a social disease that needed a social cure."[70]

The first diet book to unite detox and the new food movement was *The Great American Detox Diet* in 2005, a gourmet vegan diet book whose title alone points toward the united American detox endeavor. Vegan chef Alexandra Jamieson published *The Great American Detox Diet* after appearing as Morgan Spurlock's girlfriend in the blockbuster 2004 documentary *Super Size Me*. The documentary followed Spurlock as he embarked on an experiment to eat only McDonald's meals for thirty days. His decline was dramatic: his cholesterol shot up, he gained twenty-four pounds, and he suffered from headaches, lethargy, and sexual dysfunction. Later nominated for an Academy Award, *Super Size Me* grossed over $20 million in theaters and soon made its way into book clubs and classrooms across the nation.

If *Super Size Me* helped mainstream food politics, *The Great American Detox Diet* reintroduced the detox diet into these increasingly political discussions of food, obesity, and public health in the United States. Jamieson wrote the book to rehabilitate Spurlock and save the health of the nation. By 2005, the concept of a "diet" may have seemed faddish, fake, and decidedly antifeminist. "Using the word *diet* only brings on anxiety," Jamieson explains in her chapter titled "Why Americans Need to Detox—Not Diet." But detox diets offered a glamorous, political air to an emerging food movement that grew from upper-class political traditions of epicureanism and consumer food movements. *The Great American Detox Diet* was the first of many detox diets to combine gourmet foods with liberal politics, shaping and being shaped by the growing alternative food movement. Jamieson explicitly disavowed the legacy of addiction in detox diets, instead focusing on obesity, politics, and contemporary environmental problems.[71]

Jamieson narrates a nostalgic food history, beginning with "There was a time, of course, before the Industrial Revolution and the birth of the modern food industry . . . when we did eat whole foods." Today, "many of us have simply forgotten how to eat right." The Standard American Diet made America the "fattest nation on the planet" and is "now killing us." Modern foods are "void of natural energy," "seriously corrupt the digestive system," and are products of "huge food conglomerates [who] have a stranglehold on our consumption."[72] Jamieson's stricter, gourmet diet resists industrial foods and her recipes are a far cry from Merla Zellerbach's chicken soup and Waldorf salads. Jamieson substitutes homemade ketchup, jam, and applesauce for normally store-bought staples. Complicated recipes for sun-dried tomato tapenade and bean popsicles demand a level of culinary expertise not needed in early diet recipes. A recipe for chocolate tofu whip, for example, requires a double boiler, a food processor, and a makeshift tofu sieve. A recipe for veggie burgers calls for eighteen ingredients.

Yet these complicated recipes were presented as old-fashioned and wholesome in contrast to the artificial, unseasonal, and foreign foods of the Standard American Diet. "What is it about the Standard American Diet (SAD) that is so toxic?" Jamieson asks.[73] Hydrogenated fats and highly processed foods were largely to blame, Jamieson writes, but she also called out the larger American food environment. "It's almost impossible not to eat fast food these days—airports are filled with food-chain outlets, and highway off-ramps are full of fast-food places," she explains, adding that the

media bombard Americans with unhealthy food messages. Political bickering is also to account for why "we are killing ourselves with the Standard
American Diet." She singles out "conflicting information we get from the
government, the food industry, and various special interest groups."[74]

At the same time that Jamieson offered gourmet veganism as an antidote
to the American toxic food environment and unhealthy politics, Michael
Pollan and other early leaders of the alternative food movement advocated
for new forms of ethical consumerism and agricultural reform. Unlike food
activism in the 1960s, the alternative food movement today is less focused
on specific policies such as farm labor or segregated lunch counters. Rather,
members of the alternative food movement can be commonly characterized by their attention to the industrial food environment and their commitment to fresh, local, organic, seasonal, and sustainable foods. To "vote
with your fork" is a common refrain, as alternative food activists see the
personal as inherently political and use consumer dollars to promote a vision of whole foods, real small-scale farms, and a diverse bounty of unprocessed produce. Alternative food today responds to those age-old anxieties
about the coldness and alienation of modern life by romanticizing a Jeffersonian past of small farms and a natural, authentic way of life.

Journalist and food activist Michael Pollan has been described as the
"high holy priest" of the food movement. His bestselling 2006 *The Omnivore's Dilemma: A Natural History of Four Meals* could easily be called the
food movement's bible. The book won a spot as a *New York Times* best book
of the year in 2006, as well as winning a prestigious James Beard award. In
The Omnivore's Dilemma, Pollan advances an environmental perspective
that situates food in the global food system, demonstrating how the industrial food chain is nutritionally poor and environmentally destructive. By
tracing out the long and complicated process by which food travels from
farm to fork, Pollan criticizes the notion that nutrition can reliably measure
the value of foods and regrets Americans' fragmented approach to good
food and eating. Instead, Pollan argues that food has to be understood in
its environmental context and the best foods are "real" or "whole." Pollan
has popularized an earlier term—"nutritionism"—to describe the reductive process in which industrial capitalism isolates nutrients and ignores the
original environment in which these foods are grown and harvested.

Despite making waves in the mainstream press and kindling the nascent
food movement, very little of *The Omnivore's Dilemma* was new to the world

of dieting. Detox diets like Zellerbach's were making similar claims about the toxic food environment and nutritionism years before the terms were invented, taking on an antiscience perspective by insisting only whole or real foods could recuperate older ways of healthful living. *The Great American Detox Diet* also broadened the concept of detox to include recent controversies about global health and the export of American obesity abroad, issues which would come to characterize much of the alternative food activism in the coming years.

Both in the alternative food movement and in detox diets, global health played an ever more important role in framing the decline of the American diet. Even as *The Great American Detox Diet* took a specifically national approach, Jamieson broadened her ambitions to reach global populations and stem the export of the American diet and diet-related disease overseas. Jamieson warns her readers that the "Standard American Diet is, quite tragically, rapidly becoming the Standard World Diet." Replicating many of the narratives of the Pacific Islands diets of Native innocence and Western invasion, Jamieson issued a "global wake-up call. . . . There is now hardly a corner of the globe that hasn't been invaded by the modern Western diet and its attendant 'illnesses of excess' that plague us today: diabetes, heart disease, cancer, obesity."[75]

Pollan and Jamieson both deploy the same rhetorical strategy: to frighten American consumers by tracing the path that many industrial foods travel from farm to fork. Jamieson explains that by "understanding where your food comes from," detoxers "can understand your power in the world—that *what you buy and eat matters*."[76] She peppers her readers with questions: "Do you know in what country and under what conditions your food was grown or manufactured? . . . How many hands, from beginning to end, carried your food before it got to your table? How many ingredients, chemicals, or processes were involved in bringing one strawberry to your plate in winter?" That same origin story underlies Pollan's narrative in *The Omnivore's Dilemma*. He begins the book by noting that "the best way to answer the questions we face about what to eat was to go back to the very beginning, to follow the food chains that sustain us, all the way from the earth to the plate."[77] *The Omnivore's Dilemma* asks how "humans take part in a food chain" and pulls back the veil on industrial food. Both Pollan and Jamieson believe that understanding the origins of foods will change behavior. Linking patriotism to consumer power, Jamieson claims that "your power as a consumer is strong," adding that "since being a citizen is so closely linked with being a consumer, do your patriotic duty and get to know your food."[78]

Pollan and Jamieson reiterate "knowledge is power," a common adage in the food movement, but the relationship between knowledge and power is obscure in arguments like these. What does getting to know your food do to reform the food system? Increased knowledge rarely translates into actual change, even on an individual consumer level. In fact, the USDA Nutrition Evidence Library concluded that nutritional information on menus did little to change how diners selected or ate their meals, even when they were trying to monitor intake.[79] Judging from this analysis of diet books, many dieters may have good reason to bypass diet information for some notion of an embedded instinct.[80] When Eden dieters traded their worldly appetites—their knowledge of good and bad foods, of when and where and what to eat—for the instinctual desires of a natural hunger, the dieters relied on the God-given instincts of the body. They sidestepped the mind and consciousness altogether. Many foodies deploy a similar argument for a political end: ethically sourced, organic, local, sustainable, or real foods should somehow appeal to the palate in ways that other foods do not. "Real food tastes better than fake food," one real foods enthusiast explains after being repulsed by store-bought cookies.[81] If you have the right palate, then the right foods will taste good; the pleasures of the palate will be self-legitimating, perhaps using taste to naturalize moral and ethical evaluations of good and bad foods.

Cynics could easily turn these kinds of arguments around to accuse Jamieson, Pollan, and their ilk of epicureanism that uses easy politics to legitimate gourmet pleasures and assuage troubled consciences. Ethical consumerism is not without its critics; geographer Julie Guthman, sociologist Josée Johnston, and others have pointed out that "citizen-consumers" who protest with their dollars and vote with their forks often do little to address real-world problems.[82] Unlike the 1960s Delano grape boycott's legacy of food boycotts, today's ethical food consumerism actually legitimates choice as a marker of identity and status. To eat ethically today requires more cultural capital and a heightened sense of status and fashion and, for many critics, this sensibility smacks of elitism. As one 2010 *The Atlantic* article opened the debate about "upper-crust, arugula-laden" foodie elitism: "Is sustainable food nothing more than the lifestyle of the rich and farmers'-market loving?"[83]

These cynics have a point. But the legacy of the diet book (especially detox diets) can defend the alternative food movement against such accusations. True, Pollan and Jamieson might seem naïve or misguided to claim that knowledge is power when it comes to actual issues of food politics. Yet perhaps we should situate these claims in the longer traditions of wishful thinking in self-help and diet books. If we contextualize the alternative food movement today in the complex history of politically informed diets like detox, a more sympathetic picture emerges of today's FLOSS movement. Instead of holding Pollan to the standards of a political activist, we could compare him to Merla Zellerbach, Francis Lappé, and others who combine dietary advice with political and environmental perspectives. By looking closely at the legacy of detox diets in the United States, *The Omnivore's Dilemma* seems more like the continued politicization of the diet book rather than a new and different type of food manifesto.

Self-help traditions were also particularly relevant to the time in which Jamieson and Pollan were writing. In 2006, a self-help book called *The Secret* was featured on *The Oprah Winfrey Show* and catapulted to the top of *The New York Times* bestseller list, staying there for 146 weeks and selling nineteen million copies.[84] *The Secret* revived older self-help traditions of wishful thinking first introduced in the nineteenth century by the New Thought Movement, which alleged that humans had god-like powers and thought itself was creative.[85] Pure or optimistic thinking could create positive outcomes, just as pessimistic thinking generated negative realities. *The Secret* is an obvious heir to New Thought and today the so-called "law of attraction" explains the creative power of thinking by karmic frequency. Visualization is key to this process: if people believe they will be rich, visualize their wealth, and open their lives to newfound prosperity, they will generate a frequency that resonates into the world and, quite possibly, delivers wealth to the wishful thinkers.

The law of attraction might sound like gibberish but *The Secret* held a firm grip on believers and many of the underlying ideas leaked broadly into American culture. Jamieson called negative thoughts "toxic thinking" and urges readers to imagine positive solutions to life's problems because "very little is usually keeping us from reaching our goals if we can train our minds to stay on a positive track."[86] Even if Michael Pollan's foodies pooh-poohed the self-help of *The Secret*, no doubt many were aware of the bestseller and the underlying principles of positive thinking that have resonated so strongly with the American people for over two centuries.[87]

Foodie elitism was also a common trope when Barack Obama was ridiculed for his wince-inducing "arugula gaffe" in 2007. While campaigning in an Iowa cornfield, Obama tried to relate to rural farmers by complaining about the steep price of arugula at Whole Foods. A conservative reporting on the "arugula gap" called him a prig, an out of touch moralizer, a "white teacup, pinkie-in-the-air sort" to assume Iowa farmers paid a premium for the bitter salad green.[88] Soon after Obama won the presidency, Michael Pollan published "An Open Letter to the Next Farmer in Chief" in *The New York Times*. Pollan asked Obama to make food policy a national priority, partially because the "health of a nation's food system is a critical issue of national security."[89] Michelle Obama's Let's Move campaign took up some of these food and nutrition-related issues to stem rising rates of childhood obesity; at the time of Obama's election, around sixty-six million American children were overweight or obese.[90] She also planted a garden of spinach, fennel, and chard on the White House lawns. All across the country, the food movement grew quickly. The number of farmers' markets more than doubled between 2004 and 2014 and the sale of organics soared. In fact, the annual growth of organic food sales peaked in the years between 2005 and 2007 and they have continued to rise steadily in every year since. Organic food sales in 2012 were $28 billion and crossed the $40-billion mark in 2016.[91]

With the rise of the food movement and increasing public concern about the obesity epidemic and sustainability, detox diets have matured in the last ten years. Environmentalism, food addiction, and the toxic food environment remained staples of many detox diets, but the detox market segmented as it grew. Some, like *The Pesticide Detox* (2012) or *Sugar Detox Formula: The Perfect Diet to Beat Sugar Addiction and Cravings Naturally* (2014) are obvious descendants of earlier emphases on environmentalism or addiction. However, detox has also become a poignant symbol for the excesses of the toxic modern environment. Much as addiction came to mean more than drugs and alcohol in the 1980s, detox has become an apt metaphor for cleansing the various addictive ills of modern life from the body.

Of the weight loss diets, Woodson Merrell's 2013 *The Detox Prescription* is representative. It dedicates nearly 350 pages of case studies, testimonials, light science, and recipes to the detoxification cause. Like Zellerbach, Merrell moves between worlds. Merrell is at the fringes of respectability, educated at Columbia and a longtime Manhattan internal medicine specialist. He was the founding executive director of the Center for Health and Healing in New York and a founding member of the Consortium of Academic Health Centers for Integrative Medicine, both organizations that Quackwatch views "with considerable distrust."[92] In the world of celebrity doctors, Merrell is definitely not as famous as Dr. Oz or Mark Hyman, but he is famous enough to be blurbed by them. Hyman called the book "game-changing" and Oz called it "smart"—not high praise, necessarily, but Merrell made sure to feature the blurbs prominently on the back cover. Merrell's celebrity endorsers are Richard Gere and Donna Karan—not Bill Clinton or Beyoncé Knowles by a long shot, but famous enough.

If Merrell is a middle-of-the-road detox doctor, then *The Detox Prescription* is a centrist detox diet that promises, like most do, "weight loss, glowing skin, abundant energy, clear mind, and solid health."[93] The book might have been a bestseller but it's definitely not a game-changer, regardless of what Hyman said on the back cover. At the surface, the diet is a short-term cleanse that eliminates the usual suspects of sugary or processed foods, alcohol, and wheat. The three-day turbo cleanse consists entirely of liquids, mainly green drinks of juiced kale, spinach, and broccoli. In an echo of nineteenth-century Fletcherism, Merrell advises dieters to chew their juices—"bite down on them, roll them around in your mouth," he writes, "chew, chew, chew." Dieters drink (or, better yet, chew) green liquids in the morning, nut milks as a midmorning snack, and red and yellow-orange juices at midday. Dinner is much the same. This repeats for three days.

Just as Zellerbach broadened the drug and alcohol detoxification framework to include foods like wheat or dairy, Merrell employs a capacious definition of toxins that contains states of mind. Specific emotions or feelings are toxic triggers, including stress, anxiety, and overwork. Merrell offers specific mind/body detox plans that include instructions to gaze at a candle, make your own mantra, or practice random acts of kindness, which he abbreviates as RAOK.[94] One RAOK is to give a quarter to a kindly looking panhandler.

Modern life makes Americans sick. Merrell profiles a typical day of a typical American—"pasty, bloated, tired"—who works harder than ever, "running 100 miles an hour on scant fumes, stepping on the stress accelerator." Stress doesn't stay in the office and these Americans come home "fraught with worry" and stay up late into the night watching television, surfing the internet, or skimming Facebook. Gravely, Merrell concludes that "they are all suffering from the same pervasive, insidious disease: modern American life." Merrell only mentions addiction when he describes new technologies, worrying that "digital feeds can become a real addiction—you might not even realize how wired you really are, between your computer, mobile phone, and iPad."[95]

Without apology, Merrell revives older late-nineteenth-century gendered discourses about intellectual life and engagement in the public sphere. Merrell cautions working women about the health repercussions of ambition. Merrill recalls a few memorable cases from his practice. Poor Leila was a bloated, wheat-sensitive movie actress with box-office power. Celeste was an ambitious "workhorse" who "because she was both ambitious and driven . . . worked in overdrive all the time" and developed debilitating migraines. Migraine headaches, Merrell explains, were just one manifestation of the many toxic ways that Celeste's body was "balking at the workload."[96]

Mara's case is particularly memorable. Her case history is titled "Type-A Wonder Woman" and Merrell describes her as a real go-getter, a high-powered attorney who was just as ruthless in her legal practice as she was with her children. Merrell spares no stereotype as he calls her a tiger mom, a taskmaster, and a control freak. After "busting through the seams of her immaculately tailored designer suits," Mara comes to Merrell, frantic to lose ten pounds. While not technically overweight yet, Mara found herself "frustrated and desperate." Taking stock of this ambitious career woman, Merrell told Mara to sleep more, exercise less, and drink juice. Mara slept more, mellowed her exercise routine, drank juice for three days, and, "aha! . . . the lightbulb went on." Mara lost the weight.

Merrell's advice that women should relax, calm down, go to bed earlier, and sleep in later is all too familiar in the larger, longer discussions of women's health in the United States. Nineteenth-century neurasthenic women were similarly prescribed the "rest cure" of bed rest, relaxation, massage, and a special diet as cures for the dangers of intellectual activity and overwork. Women's health was considered particularly vulnerable to nervousness, hysteria, and other maladies in an increasingly complicated modern world. Charlotte Perkins Gilman, feminist author and activist, wrote about her experience after the famous Silas Weir Mitchell prescribed the rest cure in the haunting short story *The Yellow Wallpaper*. Along with rest and sleep, Gilman and thousands of other women prescribed the cure were massaged, overfed, and kept as motionless as possible for weeks on end.[97] Feminist scholar Gail Bederman suggests that Mitchell's rest cure infantilized increasingly strong women by prescribing a retreat from work and an "intellectually stressful civilization."[98] The cure for worldly ambition was complete domestic isolation. For both Mara and Gilman, ambition and success came at the cost of their health. Detox and the rest cure both responded to a changing, complex modern world by advising Americans to step back from civilization, relax, and allow the body to repair itself, on its own time.

Merrell's book pays its debts to political and environmental activism. In a section titled "Eating Clean Can [Help] Save the Planet," Merrell declares that "in setting out to write this book, I intend to change the planet, one life at a time."[99] Wishful thinking is critical to the weight loss endeavor, Merrell explains. Dieters must think carefully about their eating because he claims the "digestive process begins with the *mere thought* of a good meal." By controlling our minds, we better train our bodies to salivate for healthy foods and eventually lose weight. As with many contemporary detoxes, Merrell offers meditation, visualization, and other mind-body techniques to structure thought and mold reality. He explains that "of all the lifestyle changes you can make, the single most powerful is gaining control of your mind." He reiterates that "the mind is the most powerful healing tool you have. Period." To this end, he includes instructions for the following mind-control techniques: walking meditation, mantra repetition, breathing procedures, thought clearing, visualization, mindful eating, and candle gazing.[100]

It is nearly as easy to dismiss Merrell's candle gazing or Jamieson's chocolate tofu whip as *The Secret's* wishful thinking. These small, sad acts smack of powerlessness and retreat: of people who could be picketing or voting or getting angry in public instead of spending their time staring at candles or whipping tofu or wishing for a better life. Staring at a candle will never, ever change the world. And it's disingenuous of people like Merrell to suggest that it ever will. But perhaps we shouldn't see these diets as substitutes for political action but instead recast them as the stories—those deep, underlying narratives of American history—that have given food politics their power over the past forty years.

Like other powerful and enduring myths in American culture, the detoxification myth is utopian and optimistic, offering hope for a better body and a better world. Our country might be toxic, our landscape congested with ugly drive-thrus, our bodies full of greasy preservatives, but with enough thought and hopefully some action, Americans can clear out the clogs and clean up our country. Detoxification diets revive that essential American promise of infinite perfectibility of self and nation. The discourses of toxicity create a beautiful, wistful vision of history and reveal how many Americans have dreamt of health and purity in a world too often seen as sick and ugly and sad.

True, these diets might be nothing more than dreams and stories and the ineffective, gauzy stuff of myth. Yet myth is often more powerful than public policy. The stories they tell shape whole philosophies about the world and our place in it, the right course of this civilization, and what the future should hold. In many ways, however obliquely, we may come to thank detox books for the political stories that drove the organic industry, planted a vegetable garden on the White House lawns, and, perhaps, who knows, might even make good on Merrell's promise to save the world.

CONCLUSION

DIET BOOKS ARE powerful—they shape philosophies, drive industries, change lives—but the story they tell is not special. They recount the foundational myth of American culture: that of the American Adam at the brink of history—competent, innocent, ready to remake the world anew. Emerson celebrated this image in 1833, calling the American the "plain old Adam, the simple genuine self against the whole world."[1] Even back then, this was a dream. No land was new; no people could be cleansed of history. But the pains of truth only suggest the power of fiction.

Every diet book is a powerful fiction that instructs, retelling age-old myths to live by, meal-by-meal, day-by-day. They recount the narrative backbone of American culture—that familiar story of the Fall of Man and the fall of a once-blessed nation. Even if a dieter never loses weight, the continued popularity of the diet book story reveals how Americans are willing to work and ready to hope. Following a diet means plotting yourself into a shared dream to remake a lost world—and make it better this time around.

This book has charted an imaginary chronology of human origins, beginning with the many Paleolithic diets published since the mid-1970s. Paleo diets remember a simpler, innocent society when our Paleolithic ancestors lived in health and harmony. The deep-historical view of human health positions today's dieter as both a fulcrum and a fossil: an all-important hinge between past and future that demonstrates the tenacity of the human race. Paleo diets build their promises to recapture "our natural birthright of health" into a larger dream of recouping an entire healthful worldview that produced such community, leisure, and beauty.[2]

One stage closer on the imaginary timeline of human origins, Eden dieters remember the times before the Fall, evoking a prelapsarian world living and eating in God's grace. Many devotional diets share mainstream millennial rhetoric warning that obesity and diabetes will cripple the American people. But these modern jeremiads remember that "God gave Adam and Eve, and all of mankind who would follow, the ideal way to nourish their marvelous physical bodies."[3] All dieters need to do is uncover and follow that ideal set by God's grace in the Garden of Eden.

Precolonial diets recast this familiar narrative by counting colonial encounter as the expulsion, and painting the entrance into modern life as soon-fatal trauma. Pacific Islanders in particular now suffer from some of the highest rates of obesity in the world and the diets urge return—to "go back" before Western contact to when Islanders "lived in harmony with the universe."[4] Detoxification diets similarly remember a time before toxins seeped into American land and food. Detoxers believe that toxic, pesticide-laden, and processed food has warped American appetites, causing not only obesity but a host of cancers and other noncommunicable diseases. Detoxers urge a return to a more natural landscape, regulated by the principles of nature and not the hubris of man. Together all these diet books—Paleo, Eden, primitive, and detox—ask fundamental questions about civilization and disease, the past and the future. Or, to borrow the words of the 1975 *Stone Age Diet*, these diets raise questions: Who are we? Where do we come from? And where do we go from here?

Today, dieting seems embedded in American culture as a powerful part of a national consciousness built on hope and the quest for infinite perfectibility. But we are at a pivotal time. Despite decades of faithful dieting—fat-free, sugar-free, low-carb, high-carb—American obesity rates have not fallen. More than two-thirds of adults are now classified as overweight or obese.

Many believe that dieting has defrauded the American people. Diet food sales have been declining precipitously for over a decade. In fact, one market research firm found Americans were deeply suspicious of the food industry generally, and diet food in particular. Even if they followed health or wellness plans, 94 percent of respondents did not consider themselves "dieters," and more than three-quarters doubted the health claims of diet foods.[5]

"The Diet Is Dead," a woman's magazine declared in 2016.[6] Very few Americans today admit to adhering to a strict breakfast-lunch-dinner diet meal plan. The pursuit of a "healthy lifestyle" has taken dieting's place. Objective, external methods of regulation like calorie counting, points calculations, and food scales are out; subjective, internal programs for self-control have taken their place. Health-seekers are looking for "wellness plans" or "healthy lifestyle changes." Keywords include body diversity, active lifestyle, holistic, healthy, natural, fresh, and sustainable. Feminist and body diversity activists helped reshape the language of dieting. The 2016 election coverage of Donald Trump's insults against a former Miss Universe introduced concepts of "body positivity" and "fat-shaming" into mainstream American discourse. Voluptuous celebrities like the Kardashian sisters and Nicki Minaj have used images of their bodies to empower women and campaign against slut-shaming. Khloé Kardashian summarized it in her 2015 self-help and exercise book: "If there's one final thing I want to say about food, it's this: Don't diet," she warns. "I mean, the word *die* is in there!" Instead "make smart lifestyle changes" and make her recipes for cauliflower magic mash-up, Koko's kale salad, or infused water.[7]

The American Psychiatric Association is now warning of a new eating disorder: orthorexia, defined as a "pathological obsession with proper nutrition" and "clean or healthy" foods. Unlike anorexics who hide disordered eating habits, orthorexics flaunt their healthy diets, especially on social media sites and food blogs.[8] Compulsive exercise or "anorexia athletica" often accompanies orthorexia. Lifestyle plans trade one set of standards for another, even more demanding plan for toned bodies; or, as a new fitness motto says it, "Strong is the new skinny." Another fear is "skinny-fat," a new term that describes a woman who "might look good in clothes," but will "still be jiggly and even have cellulite" underneath.[9] Recent books like *Fit Is the New Skinny* (2012), *Strong Is the New Skinny* (2014), or *Strong Is the New Sexy* (2015) ask women for twice as much: being strong, sexy, healthy, and somehow intuitive enough to figure it all out on your own.

Ragging on diets is hardly new. Many dieters found it difficult to reconcile dieting and feminism in the 1960s and 70s and some authors sidestepped the issue by assuring women they weren't dieting or practicing self-denial but rather embracing health. Some such as the 1970 *New No Willpower Diet* even assured women "for the first time in your life, *you'll be dieting without feeling like a dieter.*"[10] Even the strictest diets published since the mid-1990s regularly disavow the word "diet," instead insisting that this diet is different from the rest—it will remake your body, revolutionize your relationship with food, change your life. Diet leaders act much like American writers at large, as literary scholar Shelley Fisher Fishkin has noted, "to write as if no one had ever written a work of fiction before them." Diet writers reject forebearers, coin new terminology, and claim to be new and different, often while they replicate formulaic narratives and unoriginal food plans.[11] Contemporary diets distance themselves from their predecessors by insisting they are lifestyle plans, "live-its," health manuals, or wellness programs. In many ways, healthy living and an active lifestyle are more than merely euphemisms for dieting. They also reveal aspects of dieting that were once undercover—that diets have always provided a lifestyle change, a makeover of pantry, plate, body, mind, and politics. Diets have long had these bigger ambitions; the "healthy lifestyle change" rhetoric just brings that history to light.

Dieting today may not be as easy to classify as the cut-and-dried pork chop or cabbage soup diets popular in the 1920s or Weight Watchers plans popular in the 1970s. But, in many ways, the amorphousness of dieting or health philosophies today make the project that much more interesting—instead of finding these worldviews tucked into the covers of a book, we must be more sensitive to the ubiquity of the worldviews that color our discussions about health, food, and the future of this country.

Healthy eating or lifestyle plans might also signal the maturation of an earlier diet philosophy by shifting control from diet to dieter. Julie Guthman's analysis of "healthism" shows how Americans have "cloaked their displeasure with the aesthetics of fat bodies" by using health, rather than beauty, to justify dieting and weight control.[12] A step further, sociologist Gwen Chapman explains that the "healthy eating discourse still bears evidence of disciplinary power," precisely because "external regulation" has been substituted for "greater self-regulation and self-monitoring."[13] Current trends in intuitive eating and dieting best sum up current attitudes toward healthy living. A pamphlet circulated by the Center for Mindful Eating explains that mindful eating "helps you shift the locus of control from external authorities to your body's inner wisdom."[14] In an echo of earlier traditions of positive thinking, mindfulness dieters also privilege knowledge, naturalizing the processes by which dieters are expected to know how to conform to unwritten standards. Guthman explains that these amorphous health goals are particularly difficult because, unlike a desired weight, "health can never be achieved once and for all, it requires constant vigilance in monitoring and constant effort in enhancing."[15]

When alternative food politics and weight control are brought together, the task is especially daunting. Subjective categories of food—real, natural, whole, and healthy—now characterize the contemporary food movement and diet books alike. The instruction to "eat real foods" has popped up in more than 100 diet books published in the last five years, especially foreboding in titles such as *Eat Real Food Or Else* (2016) or *Real Food, Fake Food* (2016). Thousands of food products are marketed as natural, a label the FDA has so far declined to regulate despite recommendations from consumer health groups. More difficult is the common refrain to "know where your food comes from," as in the Know Your Farmer, Know Your Food program funded by the United States Department of Agriculture in 2009. What does knowledge do, exactly? By advocating for understanding and insisting that knowledge is power, food activists today risk taking action out of the equation, instead assuming that, as good citizens, Americans should know better.

When a dieter cheats on Atkins with a Snickers, he is rebelling against external authority; when a health-conscious foodie activist cheats on his own healthy lifestyle with a Snickers, he may gnaw into his sense of self-control and his moral stance on the environment, ethics, animal cruelty, and labor. And, more important, when that foodie activist is categorized as overweight, his own body might out him, providing material proof of his weak convictions.

The capaciousness of the new mainstream politics and ubiquitous pursuit of a "healthy lifestyle" help reveal the bigger forces at stake in the future of American food, diet, and health: large food companies, developments in obesity treatment, media and celebrity, the alternative food movement, and American nutrition policy. Food companies are bellwethers of American diet trends and, as one industry expert observed in 2015, "Diet has become a forbidden four-letter word in the food industry."[16] In the past few years, fast food and commercial weight loss plans have faced similar slowdowns in sales, illustrating the two cultural shifts toward healthy and politically palatable foods. Profits of two seemingly invincible companies—Weight Watchers and McDonald's—have been declining for years. Both are afflicted by the same consumer trend: health-conscious consumers now prefer less processed foods they consider healthier and more authentic. No number of McDonald's kale salad bowls (now served at some California locations) have helped the fast food chain shed its reputation for unhealthy burgers and nuggets. Chains like Chipotle, Panda Express, and Panera Bread have seized this market share. *The Washington Post* even called the decline of fast food and rise of fast-casual restaurants the "Chipotle effect," or the new consumer demand for food quality, freshness, sustainability, and transparency.[17] However, more is at stake for food businesses built on softer appeals to ethics or health; Chipotle sales dropped nearly 30 percent in the first quarter of 2016, largely due to a much-publicized norovirus outbreak that sickened hundreds in Boston.[18] Fresh, locally sourced ingredients complicate an already complicated food safety chain and more in-house food prep means more opportunities for sick employees to spread bugs. Public agitation and unrelenting press coverage prompted Chipotle to take immediate action, shuttering all of its nearly 2,000 locations for a workday and changing food preparation methods. A year later, the business still hasn't fully recovered.

By the same token, traditional diet foods and commercial weight loss plans have seen sales suffer. Once the mainstay of the market, Weight Watchers membership has dropped even though the company claims it still has 3.6 million members.[19] Even with Oprah Winfrey's endorsement, Weight Watchers doesn't have the health aura driving so many diet books today. The company seems like it's made up of faddish fuddy-duddy housewives looking to squeeze into their little black dresses. Today, dieters look to strong, lean, and healthy plans that talk about wholeness and sustainability—not fiber points or low-calorie baking substitutes. Weight Watchers frozen entree lines can't shake the TV dinner aura. Despite the success of meal-replacement Soylent drink powder, SlimFast smoothies and Weight Watcher's meal-replacement drinks have declined in popularity. In fact, the whole frozen food market has flagged, especially individual Lean Cuisine and Weight Watchers dinners, served in tidy compartments on plastic trays.

In just one year, Lean Cuisine's meal sales fell 15 percent, costing the company $100 million.[20] Diet bars, frozen meals, shakes, pills, and programs have all seen sales drop in the last five years. Even sugar substitutes—the most common diet aids in the United States—came under fire after rumors of their carcinogenic properties appear to have been confirmed by a prominent Italian cancer researcher in 2007.[21]

All these business trends suggest a mass consumer distrust in the food status quo, or what food guru Michael Pollan described as "nutritionism" in 2007, originally coined by the Australian sociologist Gyorgy Scrinis as the "nutritionally reductive approach to food" promoted by the expansion of nutrition science and public health over the twentieth century.[22] In the last decade, both alternative food leaders and diet gurus have insisted that calorie counting and other objective measures should be traded in for subjective criteria of instinct and pleasure. Pollan considers "nutritionism" to be the post–World War I food industry orthodoxy that isolates certain properties of foods—calories, vitamins, fiber grams—and evaluates them as good or bad foods. Instead of this reductive nutrition that neglects the sum for the parts, Pollan recommends a whole and organic approach to foods, trading in Fruit Loops for fruit and soy protein isolates for beef. Jessica Mudry dates a version of nutritionism to the chemist William Atwater's late nineteenth-century calorie experiments that transformed food and eating away from the immediate "sensation of taste" and toward a more instrumental view of food energy—a shift away from "nature" to "science" as the most apt gauge of value.[23] Religious diet reformers were fighting rationalized, quantified approaches even before Atwater introduced the calorie—think back to John Harvey Kellogg's campaign against "unbiologic" living—but the alternative food movement today has revived the fundamental clash between nature and science with particular fervor.

Contemporary antinutritionism signals the mainstreaming of the alternative food movement that first gained traction in the hippie, ecological approach to whole foods in the 1960s, reviving what Rachel Laudan calls the "agrarian-romantic vision of culinary history."[24] When he issued his six food rules in *Time* in 2006, Pollan instructed Americans: "Don't eat anything your great-great-great grandmother wouldn't recognize as food." He continued by telling readers to "spend more, eat less," disregard nutritional science, and "eat with pleasure. The more I learn about the science of nutrition, the less certain I am that we've learned anything important about food that our ancestors didn't know," he explains.[25] At its core, Pollan's philosophy is a rejection of modern nutrition science and privileges the shapeless qualities of instinct, common sense, and pleasure. Like mindful eaters, Pollan wrests control away from top-down authorities to give it back to the individual eater. Earlier diet books promoted similar philosophies, but now that eater is held to perhaps even stricter external standards: don't be fat, eat ethically, reject the agricultural-industrial complex, and savor every mouthful all the while.

At the same time the food movement has shifted away from careful, scientific measurement of calories and carbs in diet plans, obesity researchers are developing promising new treatments. Many health-seekers today both denounce science-based nutritionism and eagerly wait for new drug development and obesity research. Despite these antiscience shifts, obesity treatments and bariatric medicine have improved rapidly over the last decade. In January 2015, the Federal Food and Drug Administration (FDA) issued the first approval for an obesity treatment device in over a decade—called the Maestro Rechargeable System, it uses an important new "electroceutical" called vBloc. Unlike older gastric bands that tie off the stomach, vBloc generates electrical pulses via electrodes.[26] The FDA also approved four different weight loss drugs between 2012 and 2014; many others are in the pipeline. All four drugs work to decrease appetite by suppressing the hunger signals transmitted to the brain. In both instinctive dieting and these new obesity drugs, the brain is bypassed, reworking the rational calculations of nutrition and relying instead on hunger (however manipulated by appetite suppressants). One of the most promising, Belviq, belongs to a class of drugs called selective serotonin reuptake inhibitors, most commonly used in treating depression and mood disorders. Belviq treats obesity by quelling the urge to eat.

None of these drugs or devices are silver bullets, but the fanfare generated by each FDA approval demonstrates how desperately the public wants an effective and safe obesity treatment. The history of obesity treatment is littered with horrific unintended consequences—the fen-phen deaths in the 1980s most immediately come to mind—but these new medical developments do show promise. Science and technology have also shaped American dieting on the micro scale. The explosive popularity of meal-tracking apps and activity trackers have given ordinary people granular data about their eating and exercise. Wearable technologies like the Fitbit Tracker measure data like step count, heart rate, sleep quality, and calories burned. Though older devices like pedometers and heart rate monitors provided this information before the mid-2000s, the 2007 Fitbit was the first wearable wireless-connected device to gain mass appeal. From 2007 to 2015, Fitbit estimates that the company sold more than twenty million of these devices. Nearly eleven million were sold in 2014 alone. MyFitnessPal, the nutrition and fitness tracking app, has enrolled forty million users.[27] Though not necessarily weight loss aids, wearable technologies demonstrate the public's eagerness to improve their diet and health. Many new diet books also incorporate wearable technologies and online calorie-counting aids.

Wearable technologies represent a gender shift in the world of dieting by taking a masculine approach to "health-tracking" that purposefully distances itself from dieting. Far more men are prominent in American food and dieting today, especially in high-profile media. One tech expert has observed that dieting has migrated into the "male-dominated startup scene," with groups of men issuing weekly tweets of their weight. "By combining tech trends like GPS, gamification, the data-driven self-help of 'the quantified self,' and old-fashioned oversharing, weight loss has become just another chore in need of hacking," the expert notes.[28]

Nothing could have signaled a cultural shift more clearly than when young, fit men entered the world of American dieting in the early 2000s. Dieting might still evoke fussy housewives, but "healthy lifestyle" and "food revolution" are terms now tied to forward-thinking, fit men such as Jamie Oliver, Anthony Bordain, Eric Schlosser, and Morgan Spurlock.[29] Historically, male diet book authors have often used the same autobiographical, empathetic narratives as their female counterparts. Today, more male diet book authors strut their own good health to inspire their readers, perhaps because the assumption is that now everyone, even thin people, must resist the spread of the obesity epidemic.

Thirty-three-year-old San Francisco–based Tim Ferris brought young men into the fold with his 2010 hit book *The 4-Hour Body: An Uncommon Guide to Rapid Fat-Loss, Incredible Sex, and Becoming Superhuman*. Ferris distanced himself from doctors and dieters alike with his tech hacker persona, calling himself a "meticulous data cruncher" who used his own body as a "laboratory of one."[30] Recalling Vilhjalmur Stefansson's all-meat experiment, others have used their bodies as "laboratories" to test out the deleterious effects of food. Most famously, Morgan Spurlock was thirty-two when he produced *Super Size Me*, the documentary film that chronicled his McDonald's-only diet experiment.

On TV, thirty-five-year-old Jamie Oliver's surprising hit—*Food Revolution*—drew international attention to the poor quality of American school lunch meals. The show followed Oliver, a British chef, across the United States as he taught townsfolk about healthy nutrition. He began in Huntington, West Virginia, in 2011—a town that was then and is still among the country's most overweight cities. Anthony Bourdain, another celebrity chef, is famous as a swaggering bad boy of the rough-and-tumble food world. As one food critic notes in her 2012 "When Meals Get Macho" article in the *New Yorker*, "Anthony Bourdain turn[ed] my good, plain meals into a demonstration of virility. . . . In the land of Bourdain, no dinner is complete without stentorian grunting, cursing, and beating one's chest."[31]

Cooking shows and food programming like Bourdain's offer an indisputable picture of the profound changes in American food culture over the last decade. Just as Julia Child democratized haute cuisine in the 1960s, celebrity chefs of the early 2000s dramatized cooking on what one food studies scholar calls a highly theatrical "performative platform."[32] Men dominate new food TV: Emeril Lagasse, Bobby Flay, Al Roker, and the many Iron Chefs. Some call these new shows "food porn," or, more recently, "gastro-porn." Instead of Julia Child's vision of a fallible, relatable domesticity, new high-production shows like *Iron Chef, Chopped, MasterChef, Hell's Kitchen, Ramsay's Kitchen Nightmares*, or *Cutthroat Kitchen* sensationalize cooking, filling the process with sharp knives, cuss words, and fierce competition.

Celebrity diet doctors are also more likely to be men. Mark Hyman has averaged about a book a year since 2005, including titles such as *Ultra-Prevention, Ultra-Metabolism, UltraSimple Diet, The Blood Sugar Solution*, and *Eat Fat, Get Thin*. Mehmet Oz (Dr. Oz) and Phil McGraw (Dr. Phil) both used their wildly popular talk shows to launch diet book empires. Dr. Oz began cowriting the You series (*You on a Diet, You Being Beautiful, You: The Owner's Manual*) in 2006; Dr. Phil published his first diet book, *The Ultimate Weight Solution*, the same year.

Higher education has taken notice of all this activity. Food studies degree-granting programs have popped up in major universities, incorporating law, business, the humanities, and clinical nutrition to bring interdisciplinary perspective to contemporary food issues. New York University offers the only PhD and includes the study of nutrition and public health under the umbrella of food studies. Other academic programs have grown from earlier gastronomic emphases: Boston University offers a masters of liberal arts in gastronomy and grants vocational certificates. In 2015, the University of the Pacific food studies master's degree program welcomed its first class in San Francisco. Clearly, these food studies degrees are as diverse as the prominent food activists and enthusiasts who have so shaped the American "foodscape" (a new buzzword in the food studies scene).

Academics prominent in these programs are also public figures. Michael Pollan is a professor of journalism at UC Berkeley; Marion Nestle holds three professorial appointments in nutrition, food studies, and public health as well as in sociology at NYU and as a visiting professor of nutritional sciences at Cornell University. Their public lectures draw huge crowds. Michael Pollan's 2006 *The Omnivore's Dilemma* and Marion Nestle's 2007 *What to Eat* both stayed on bestseller lists for months.

The distinction between "foodies" and "food activists" looks clear from 40,000 feet. Foodies are wealthy, indulgent, navel-gazing pleasure-seekers. Food activists are tireless, unpretentious warriors in the battle for farmworkers' rights, humane treatment of animals, public nutrition assistance, and environmentally responsible agriculture. On the ground, however, foodies and food activists overlap most when they unite behind a single food-related cause. In the 2009 *Foodies: Democracy and Distinction in the Gourmet Foodscape*, one of the first full-length books on the topic, scholars Josée Johnston and Shyon Baumann define the term loosely: foodies are culinary amateurs "obsessively interested in the gastronomic."[33] Unlike snobbish gourmets, foodies eat across class lines, often romanticizing ethnic "hole-in-the-wall" restaurants. Alternative food activists see the personal as inherently political and vote with their fork to use consumer dollars to promote a vision of whole foods, real small-scale farms, and a diverse bounty of unprocessed produce.

Foodies rarely rally behind large-scale political efforts like farmworkers' rights or fast-food workers' minimum wages. Rather, foodies and even some diet gurus promote products and practices that improve flavor and the eating experience. Sometimes they advance environmentalism and animal rights, especially as they affect flavor as with grass-fed beef, cage-free eggs, local foods, and organic produce. Since 2002, certified organic operations have increased by nearly 300 percent and as of 2016 there are nearly

22,000 of these operations in the United States alone. The total retail market for organic products in the United States was valued at $39 billion in 2016.[34]

Organics have moved beyond the farmers' market and Whole Foods crowd; the largest purveyor of organic food in this country is now Wal-Mart. With its recent acquisition of Whole Foods, Amazon might build in organics from the ground up in their massive push to develop online grocery shopping. Cage-free policies have passed into state law after mass consumer activism demanded the humane treatment of chickens. California Proposition 2 passed in 2008 as the "Prevention of Farm Animal Cruelty Act," requiring egg-laying hens to "be confined only in ways that allow these animals to lie down, stand up, fully extend their legs and turn around freely."[35] McDonald's has pledged to transition to cage-free eggs by 2025. The largest egg buyer in the United States, McDonald's currently serves more than two billion eggs a year and this bold decision may remake the entire egg supply chain.

Taken as a whole, this activity has significantly changed food and nutrition in the United States. In 2012, Centers for Disease Control reports began to show proof of progress: obesity rates appear to have leveled off between 2003 and 2012. Over a third of American adults and nearly a fifth of American children are classified as obese, but the upward trend has stabilized. While childhood obesity rates may have tripled since 1980, studies now show overall rates to have leveled off over the last decade.[36] Some researchers postulate that the "cumulative effect of public health programs" has stabilized childhood obesity by increasing physical activity, reducing TV watching, and cutting down on soft drinks.[37] Yet these same researchers warn that child obesity rates in developing countries continue to rise dramatically, echoing the trends seen in the developed world two or three decades before. Middle-income countries like Indonesia and Mexico now face what experts call the "double burden of malnutrition," or comparable rates of both hunger and obesity.

An odd mix of activists, religious leaders, reformers, gourmets, and dieters have fundamentally reshaped the American food system over the last hundred years. Their good efforts have shown Americans the political consequences and symbolism of food. They may have also helped stem the defining public health crisis of our time. Every action mattered—vending machine bans, soda taxes, new regulations, public awareness campaigns, mandated recesses—for these unlikely alliances to combat the rising tide of obesity in the United States. American diets and dieting have precipitated the politics of the alternative food movement, charging it with far bigger ambitions. Especially with detox, many of these diets have both interpreted and relayed radical food politics, offering an easy-to-understand set of food philosophies that has shaped public perception of larger political issues.

These developments deserve recognition but diets do more than reflect or reveal food politics. They also do more than retell that old, familiar story—the ache of the Fall of Man, the longing for home, the promise of the possible—that is the narrative backbone of our national consciousness. Diet books are the stories that people live by, eat with, believe in, and act on. They are useful fictions, more like theater than literature. They build a stage on which we play out the big dramas of mankind: God and man, sickness and health, and the success or failure of human civilization.

It's difficult to grow tired of diet books. There's a lullaby in the sameness of the story. The diet books repeat themselves, mourning the same fallen world, promising the same future, berating the same people for the same reasons: for being fat and ugly, for reneging on their promise, for being sick and sad and stressed. Paleo diets mourn our buried caveman past; devotional diets remember God's grace; primitive diets lament a paradise corrupted by colonialism; detoxification diets grieve for a virgin land now sullied by industry. Diet books may repeat themselves, but strength is to be had from steadfast insistence. We should think of diet books as a bugle, a banshee, something that calls out and insists Americans pay attention to a story—our story—that we are all writing with every meal.

And, together, the diet books show how we create a culture Clifford Geertz defined as "simply the ensemble of stories we tell ourselves about ourselves."[38] That simple chorus make these stories worthwhile—the broad, generous, young narratives that unite Americans too often divided by a tired sort of world-weariness. Maybe, just maybe, the tender hope of the diet book is proof of our willingness to do good and believe in the stories worth believing in.

ACKNOWLEDGMENTS

Diet and the Disease of Civilization is the product of untold institutional generosity and inspirational mentorship. My professors, advisors, colleagues, classmates, and family not only supported my research but also inspired my thinking and buoyed my faith. I am indebted to them and the institutions—Stanford and UC Berkeley, mainly—that continue to value the intellectual work of the humanities.

At the Schlesinger Library at the Radcliffe Institute for Advanced Study, culinary archives revealed scores of business-sponsored health advice documents and recipes. Grants awarded by the Marilyn Yalom Research Fund of the Michelle Clayman Institute for Gender Research and the Stanford Community Engagement and Vice Provost Graduate Research Opportunity programs sponsored interviews, the acquisition of a private collection, and the purchase of nontraditional research materials. Without the funding provided by the Modern Thought and Literature program at Stanford University and Mellon Foundation Dissertation Fellowship, this work would never have been conceived, much less completed. The Lane History of Science, Medicine, and Technology Grant program sponsored research that contributed to the Pacific Islands chapter.

I wish to recognize Etta Madden and Lyman Tower Sargent for editing a special edition of *Utopian Studies* on food and so providing my work with a powerful intellectual framework. A version of the Paleo chapter was published in *Utopian Studies* in 2015. Benjamin Reiss deserves much gratitude for his thorough and insightful comments on this manuscript draft. My anonymous readers also carefully reviewed this book and offered helpful critique. Interviews with dieters, public health activists, and diet book authors provided personal insight. I am grateful to Leslie Mitchner and the staff of Rutgers University Press for supervising the development of this manuscript with care and acuity. Lisa Banning, Jenny Blanc-Tal and Phoebe Keller have been infinitely patient with edits and revisions.

Very recently, Sandra Greene, Aaron Sachs, John Barwick, Joan Jacobs Brumberg, and Penny von Eschen have warmly welcomed me into the History department at Cornell University. Rosemarie Garland-Thomson helped me think through the next phase of this research. In food studies, I thank Carolyn Dimitri and Krishnendu Ray for hosting me as a visiting scholar at New York University. Enriching conversations and the Marion Nestle Food Studies Collection aided this research immensely. Ken Albala and Polly Adema at University of the Pacific invited me to discuss food fads with a talented group of food studies scholars and Alissa Merksamer welcomed me to the food world in San Francisco.

This book began with my professors at University of California, Berkeley. My research ideas took shape when Professors Moran and Lovell introduced me to American studies in September 2006. In the crowded lecture hall for "Food in America," Professor Moran lectured about an America that I thought I knew but actually was just discovering. Professor Lovell's keen eye for folk art and agile way of thinking opened me to the possibilities of artistic interpretation of everyday objects. Greil Marcus modeled the practices of cultural criticism, setting an example for intuitive, responsible, and astute analysis of music and culture.

At Stanford, many friends and classmates in modern thought and literature deserve gratitude for their support and camaraderie: Cam Awkward-Rich, Karli Cerankowski, Vanessa Chang, Alexis Charles, Maria Cichosz, Lindsey Dolich Felt, Corey Johnson, Ronmel Navas, Laura Rogers, Max Seuchting, Vasile Stanescu, and Rebecca Wilbanks. The directors of modern thought and literature—Michelle Elam, Ursula Heise, and Paula Moya—guided the program with purpose and skill. Rachel Meisels and Monica Moore always ensured the mechanics of modern thought ran smoothly. Mary Munil acquired obscure texts through interlibrary loan. Scott Bukatman, Ramon Saldívar, Kyoto Sato, Fred Turner, and Tobias Wolf provided invaluable support and academic counsel. The kind, brilliant people who make up Stanford University deserve countless thanks, but the institution itself also deserves recognition. Stanford University should be praised for its generosity and institutional commitment to art and the humanities.

My family has long encouraged these research interests and gratitude goes to Elias Goodman, Nathaniel Johnson, Lev Abraham Jacobson, Tamara Jacobson, David Ezekiel Johnson, Muriel Weintraub, and Lynn Seller. I am also grateful to the late Rita Goodman, Abraham Goodman, and Adelyn Johnson. Dena Goodman reviewed many early proposals of this book and long encouraged my academic pursuits. Daniel Goodman provided valuable insight into detoxification and the history of fasting.

Judith Goodman's commitment to education and undeterred pursuit of an advanced degree inspired me from the start. This book benefited from her careful legal perspective and its author benefited even more from her tenacity and encouragement. Thank you.

I have others to thank for their kindness and kinship: George Bitar, Janet Bitar, Vanesa Bottger, Ruth Bram, Natalie Glatzel, Phoebe Katzenbach, Anne Leicher, Zoe Maxon, Adriana Monroy, and Juliette Mrockowski. Judy and Stan Phillips's enthusiasm for my endeavors brought joy to this research over the years. Discussions with Ateeq Suria and others on the Graduate Student Council broadened my thinking to include engineering, politics, and business. I thank Summer Shafer for her comradeship in American Studies 10 and Melissa Fall for sharing her literary talents in our writing seminars.

My dissertation committee at Stanford set an example for academic inquiry, interdisciplinary creativity, and personal generosity. Bryan Wolf unearthed the layers of meaning in American art and the subtle, powerful codes of culture. Professor Wolf opened me to the possibilities of art and I saw how to see—really see—through his brilliant eyes. His analysis of Thomas Cole's *Expulsion from the Garden of Eden* and Winslow Homer's *The Morning Bell* still provide a model of intellect and empathy.

Estelle Freedman modeled an example of commitment and scholarly rigor, guiding me through the challenges of historical research with grace. Her attention to the history of women and gender analysis was critical to organizing my arguments and archive. Her sensitive, smart analysis of primary sources sets the standard for archival research. Professor Freedman's unflinching commitment to historical inquiry proved to me tenfold the values of perseverance and conviction.

Shelley Fisher Fishkin supported this book from proposal to publication. Her insights into American literature and skills of cultural analysis always sparked new ideas. My writing and thinking improved with every meeting and comment tagged in track changes. The joyfulness with which she approached the detective work of research motivated me to consider alternative viewpoints and unusual sources. Professor Fishkin never failed to inspire me with the power of her academic research and the warmth of her mentorship. I owe a great deal to her.

And I thank Eilyan Bitar for his steadfast faith and encouragement. He showed me, early on, what it means to share the joy of learning. Eilyan's work demonstrates how good research really can improve the world and he inspires me to work harder, write more, and, together, revel in the joys of education and discovery. I thank him for the gift of his love and respect.

Even as I thank all these extraordinary friends and scholars, one debt of gratitude seems impossible to articulate. I got lucky to have a talented speechwriter and newspaper reporter for a father, but was even luckier that, with patience and love, my father taught me how to write. As my lifelong editor, Michael McIntyre Johnson has read thousands of pages over the last fifteen years, correcting grammar mistakes, reordering paragraphs, chopping up long sentences, and always adding in dashes—to emphasize, of course, the strength of my claims. This one—my father, my editor—is for you.

NOTES

INTRODUCTION

1 Boston Medical Center, *Nutrition and Weight Management*, https://www.bmc.org /nutrition-and-weight-management/weight-management. Forty five million dieters is a conservative estimate, not least because many people trying to lose weight eschew the dieter identity. One 2010 report estimated upwards of ninety million dieters. Stephanie Mariko Finn explains the disparity as a difference in data measurement, but the range does suggest an even larger population than previously understood. Marketdata Enterprises, *The U.S. Weight Loss Market: 2014 Status Report & Forecast*, February 20, 2014, http://www.prnewswire.com/news-releases/the-us-weight-loss-market-2014-status -report--forecast-246304741.html; Robert S. Goldfarb, Thomas C. Leonard, and Steven Suranovic, "Modeling Alternative Motives for Dieting," *Eastern Economic Journal* 32, no. 1 (Winter 2006): 115; Centers for Disease Control, National Center for Health Statistics, *Health, United States, 2014: With Special Feature on Adults Aged 55–64* (Hyattsville, MD: CDC, 2015), 199, http://www.cdc.gov/nchs/data/hus/hus14.pdf#059; Stephanie Mariko Finn, "Aspirational Eating: Class Anxiety and the Rise of Food in Popular Culture" (PhD diss., University of Michigan, 2011), 152.

2 National Institute of Diabetes and Digestive Kidney Diseases, *Overweight and Obesity Statistics*, October 2012, https://www.niddk.nih.gov/health-information/health-statistics/overweight-obesity; Roland Sturm and Aiko Hattori, "Morbid Obesity Rates Continue to Rise Rapidly in the United States," *International Journal of Obesity* 37, no. 6 (June 2013): 889–891.

3 By body mass index (BMI), an average height man or woman would be morbidly obese if they weigh 240 or 210 pounds, respectively, and considered overweight at 174 or 146 pounds. BMI is a crude measurement tool, however, and by BMI alone, muscular athletes like Arnold Schwarzenegger and Sammy Sosa (in their prime) would be obese. George Blackburn and W. Allan Walker, "Science-Based Solutions to Obesity: What Are the Roles of Academia, Government, Industry, and Health Care?," *The American Journal of Clinical Nutrition* 82, no. 1 (July 1, 2005): 207.

4 Lee F. Monaghan, *Men and the War on Obesity: A Sociological Study* (London: Routledge, 2008), 1.

5 R.W.B. Lewis, *The American Adam: Innocence, Tragedy, and Tradition in the Nineteenth Century* (Chicago: University of Chicago Press, 1955), 3.

6 Warren Belasco, *Food: The Key Concepts* (New York: Berg, 2008), 91.

7 E. Melanie DuPuis, *Dangerous Digestion: The Politics of American Dietary Advice* (Berkeley: University of California Press, 2015), 2.

8 Food Marketing Institute, *Supermarket Facts*, https://www.fmi.org/our-research /supermarket-facts.

9 Hasia Diner, *Hungering for America: Italian, Irish, and Jewish Foodways in the Age of Migration* (Cambridge, MA: Harvard University Press, 2001), 10.

10 Katharina Vester, "Regime Change: Gender, Class, and the Invention of Dieting in Post-Bellum America," *Journal of Social History* 44, no. 1 (Fall 2010), 39.

11 Ibid.

12 Sander Gilman, "Banting, William," in *Diets and Dieting: A Cultural Encyclopedia* (New York: Routledge, 2008), 15–17.

13 Louise Foxcroft, *Calories and Corsets: A History of Dieting over Two Thousand Years* (London: Profile Books, 2011), 78–79.

14 "Corpulence," *Scientific American* 47 (November 4, 1882): 289.

15 Both Banting and Fletcher live on in contemporary dieting, inspiring the counsel to "chew, chew, chew" in the 2013 *The Detox Prescription* or recent hits such as the 2016 *The Banting Solution*. Bernadine Douglas and Bridgette Allan, *The Banting Solution: Your Low-Carb Guide to Permanent Weight Loss* (Cape Town, South Africa: Penguin, 2016); Woodson Merrell, *The Detox Prescription: Supercharge Your Health, Strip Away Pounds, and Eliminate the Toxins Within* (Emmaus, PA: Rodale Press), 99.

16 John D'Emilio and Estelle Freedman, *Intimate Matters: A History of Sexuality in America* (New York: Harper & Row, 1988), 67–68.

17 Karen Iacobbo and Michael Iacobbo, *Vegetarian America: A History* (Westport, CT: Prager, 2004), 14.

18 Kyla Wazana Tompkins, *Racial Indigestion: Eating Bodies in the 19th Century* (New York, New York University Press, 2012), 63–64.

19 Howard Markel, "John Harvey Kellogg and the Pursuit of Wellness," *Journal of the American Medical Association* 305, no. 17 (2011): 1814.

20 John Harvey Kellogg, *The Battle Creek Sanitarium System: History, Organization, Methods* (Battle Creek, MI: Gage Printing, 1908), 117.

21 Arlene Spark, Lauren Dinour, and Janel Obenchain, *Nutrition in Public Health: Principles, Policies, and Practice* (Boca Raton, FL: CRC Press, 2007), 66.

22 Ibid., 319.

23 Frank Surface and Raymond L. Bland, *American Food in the World War and Reconstruction Period: Operations of the Organizations under the Direction of Herbert Hoover, 1914 to 1924* (Stanford, CA: Stanford University Press, 1931).

24 Rima Dombrow Apple, *Vitamania: Vitamins in American Culture* (New Brunswick, NJ: Rutgers University Press, 1996), 4.

25 Bertrand M. Patenaud, *A Wealth of Ideas: Revelations from the Hoover Institution Archives* (Stanford, CA: Stanford General Books, 2006), 39.

26 Helen Zoe Veit, *Modern Food, Moral Food: Self-Control, Science, and the Rise of Modern American Eating in the Early Twentieth Century* (Chapel Hill: University of North Carolina Press, 2013), 19.

27 Ibid., 14.

28 *War-Time Cook and Health Book*, in *John W. Hartman Center for Sales, Advertising & Marketing History, Rare Book, Manuscript, and Special Collections Library*, Duke University, http://library.duke.edu/rubenstein/scriptorium/eaa/cookbooks/CK0075/CK0075 -01-72dpi.html.

29 Supposedly authored by Thompson's French-speaking female associate and alter ego known only as "Mahdah," *Eat and Grow Thin*'s cosmopolitan menus represent a combined American-European fight against fat: stewed celery, onions, fish, and other unassuming American fare were presented alongside soufflé, filet jardinière, and cantaloupe frappe. Vance Thompson, *Eat and Grow Thin: The Mahdah Menus* (New York: E. P. Dutton & Company, 1914), 12–21.

30 Rebecca Haynes, "An Appetite for Weight Loss: Americans Hooked on Unhealthy Fad Diets," *Connecticut Post*, September 27, 2010, http://www.ctpost.com/mind/article /An-Appetite-for-Weight-Loss-Americans-hooked-on-637235.php.

31 Angela Willey, "Peters, Lulu Hunt," in Gilman, *Diets and Dieting*, 211–212.

32 Lulu Hunt Peters, *Diet and Health, with Key to the Calories* (Chicago: The Reilly and Lee Co., 1918), 79.

33 Ibid., 110.

34 Peter Stearns, *Fat History: Bodies and Beauty in the Modern West* (New York: New York University Press, 1997), 124.

35 Vester, "Regime Change," 39.

36 Charles Kupfer, "Il Duce and the Father of Physical Culture," *Iron Game History* 6, no. 2 (January 2000): 3–9.

37 The word "fad" was also disavowed from the start. An 1897 editorial in the *Yorkville Enquirer* warned about the dangers of fad diets for children. With more fanfare, an anonymous source consulted for a 1911 *Washington Post* article on diet and French beauty tips explained that "the diet is not a fad diet: you can't be a faddist and succeed" on a rational plan of mayonnaise and double-cooked foods. Faddish food trends became the butt of anti-German jokes on the eve of World War I, such as the "pink bread fad" or the "blue lobster" diet. Beginning in 1913, some German chefs were tinting bread and coloring soup and, by boiling lobster in alkalinized water, serving sky blue crustaceans for the smart set of high-society Germans. "Dangers of the Diet Fad," *Yorkville Enquirer* (South Carolina), February 24, 1897, in *Chronicling America: Historic American Newspapers*, Library of Congress, http://chroniclingamerica.loc.gov/; "Eat and Remain Young, French Secret for Beauty," *The Washington Post*, January 15, 1911; "The Pink Bread Fad: The Color of Foods Believed to Be Indicative of Personal Character and Are Easily Arranged," *Los Angeles Times*, November 9, 1913.

38 Jane Calhoun, "Diet and Flesh Reduction," *Harper's Bazaar* 45, no. 12 (1911): 576.

39 Heather Addison, *Hollywood and the Rise of Physical Culture* (New York: Routledge, 2003), 41–42.

40 Amanda Regan, *"Madame Sylvia of Hollywood and Physical Culture, 1920–1940"* (MA thesis, California State University San Marcos, 2013), 58.

41 Grace Wilcox, "DIET-DIET," *Daily Boston Globe*, December 15, 1935, 8.

42 Fannie Hurst, *No Food with My Meals* (New York: Harper & Brothers, 1935), 50.

43 "Society Beauties Seek Health & Complexion in Vegetables," *Chicago Daily Tribune*, July 23, 1905.

44 "Eat and Remain Young, French Secret for Beauty," *The Washington Post*, January 15, 1911.

45 "Dangers in Diets," review of *Diet and Die* by Carl Malmberg, *The New York Times*, October 13, 1935, BR12.

46 Carole Davis and Etta Saltos, *Dietary Recommendations and How They Have Changed over Time*, in *America's Eating Habits: Changes and Consequences*, ed. E. Frazao (Washington, DC: United States Department of Agriculture, 1999), 35, http://www.ers.usda.gov/media/91022/aib750b_1_.pdf.

47 Regan, *"Madame Sylvia,"* 110.

48 Amy Bentley, *Eating for Victory: Food Rationing and the Politics of Domesticity* (Chicago: University of Illinois Press, 1998), 102–103.

49 Spark et al., *Nutrition in Public Health*, 346–347.

50 Harvey Levenstein, *Fear of Food: A History of Why We Worry about What We Eat* (Chicago: The University of Chicago Press, 2012), 140.

51 Roberto Ferdman, "The Generational Battle of Butter vs. Margarine," *The Washington Post*, June 17, 2014, https://www.washingtonpost.com/news/wonk/wp/2014/06/17/the-generational-battle-of-butter-vs-margarine/.

52 Levenstein, *Fear of Food*, 136.

53 Cubbison Cracker Company, *Cubbison's Party Guide: Slenderizing Menus and Recipes* (Los Angeles: Cubbison Cracker Co., 1933); *The Cook Book Of Glorious Eating For Weight Watchers: Recipes and Menus from Wesson to Help Prevent Overweight* (New Orleans, LA: Wesson People, 1961), in the Alan and Shirley Brocker Sliker Collection, MSS 314, Special Collections, Michigan State University Libraries.

54 Walter Alvarez, "Seeing the Doctor: Diet a Lifetime Business—Not a 10-Day Miracle," *Daily Boston Globe*, October 16, 1956, 18.

55 Some new recipes called for saccharin and cyclamates, but de la Peña also points out that individual dieters worked with the chemicals to "control and limit sugar calories" and the experimentation also provided "positive experiences such as creativity, control, and self-care." Carolyn de la Peña, *Empty Pleasures: The Story of Artificial Sweeteners from Saccharin to Splenda* (Chapel Hill: University of North Carolina Press, 2010), 39.

56 "Those Foods for Dieters," *Changing Times* 8, no. 1 (1954): 13.

57 Poppy Cannon, *Unforbidden Sweets: Delicious Desserts of 100 Calories or Less* (New York: Collier Books, 1958).

58 Bentley, *Eating for Victory*, 87.

59 Mintz, Sidney. *Sweetness and Power: The Place of Sugar in Modern History* (New York: Penguin Books, 1985), 160.

60 Carole M. Counihan, introduction to *Food and Gender: Identity and Power*, ed. Carole M. Counihan and Steven L. Kaplan (New York: Routledge, 1998), 2–3.

61 *Keeping Your Weight Down!: The Welch Way to Weight Control* (New York: The Welch Grape Juice Co., 1933), in the Alan and Shirley Brocker Sliker Collection, MSS 314, Special Collections, Michigan State University Libraries.

62 Sugar Research Foundation, *A Suggested Program for the Cane and Beet Sugar Industries*, October 1942, 1–2, https://archive.org/details/480900-a-suggested-program-for-the-cane-and-beet-sugar.

63 "It's Smart to Stay Slim and Trim and Get Domino's 'Energy Lift' Too!," *The Chicago Daily Tribune*, April 9, 1954, B8.

64 *Keep Slim And Trim with Domino Sugar Menus* (New York: American Sugar Refining Co., 1954), in the Alan and Shirley Brocker Sliker Collection, MSS 314, Special Collections, Michigan State University Libraries, 24.

65 Norman Jolliffe, *Reduce and Stay Reduced* (New York: Simon and Schuster, 1952), x, 24.

66 H. Pollack, "Reduce and Stay Reduced," *American Journal of Public Health and the Nation's Health* 42, no. 11 (1952): 1482–1483.

67 Jolliffe, 7.

68 Jane Nickerson, "News of Food: City Nutrition Expert Explains in Book How to Reduce and Stay at Right Weight," *The New York Times*, May 20, 1952, 28; Ida Jean Kain, "Maybe Your Appestat Needs Reconditioning," *The Washington Post*, August 27, 1952, 23.

69 Etta M. Madden and Martha L. Finch, *Eating in Eden: Food and American Utopias* (Lincoln: University of Nebraska Press, 2006), 163.

70 Warren J. Belasco, *Appetite for Change: How the Counterculture Took On the Food Industry* (Ithaca, NY: Cornell University Press, 1989).

71 Catherine Manton, *Fed Up: Women and Food in America* (Westport, CT: Bergin & Garvey, 1999), 67.

72 Susie Orbach, *Fat Is a Feminist Issue: The Anti-Diet Guide to Permanent Weight Loss* (New York: Paddington Press, 1978).

73 Naomi Wolf, *The Beauty Myth: How Images of Beauty Are Used against Women* (New York: W. Morrow, 1991), 187.

74 Gwen E. Chapman, "From 'Dieting' to 'Healthy Eating': An Exploration of Shifting Constructions of Eating for Weight Control," in *Interpreting Weight: The Social Management of Fatness and Thinness*, ed. Jeffrey Sobal and Donna Maurer (New York: Aldine de Gruyter, 1999), 81.

75 Vester, "Regime Change," 40.

76 Elise Paradis, "Changing Meanings of Fat: Fat, Obesity, Epidemics, and America's Children" (PhD diss., Stanford University, 2011), 52.

77 World Health Organization, *Obesity: Preventing and Managing the Global Epidemic*, Report of a WHO Consultation on Obesity (Geneva: WHO, 1998), 9.

78 Disability theorist Rosemarie Garland-Thomson has deftly shown how only a "very small minority" of people actually meet the "narrow criteria of the idealized norm." The image of a normal majority persists, however, because it is "an image that dominates without material substance, a phantom 'majority' opposed to an overwhelming and equally illusory 'minority.'" If two hundred million Americans fall outside the normal category, perhaps the deviance of a majority might lay bare structures of power, methods of oppression, and "the processes that construct both the normative and the deviant." But the thin ideal has not abated. In fact, studies show a historically inverse relationship between the size of fashion models (now a size 00) and average American women (size 14–16). By today's standards, supermodels Christie Brinkley and Cindy Crawford would likely be classified as "plus-size" models. Diet leaders often invoke a "deviant normal" framework to push Americans to quickly stem the obesity epidemic

rather than question the social frame that could stigmatize two-thirds of the population. After describing chubby kids and "muffin topped and hollow eyed" teenagers, one Paleo diet explained how "normal can be mistaken for 'common,' because the above conditions are neither right nor normal." Rosemarie Garland-Thomson, *Extraordinary Bodies: Figuring Physical Disability in American Culture and Literature* (New York: Columbia University Press, 1997), 32; Wolf, *The Paleo Solution*, 11.

79 Christine Himes, "The Demography of Obesity," in *The Oxford Handbook of the Social Science of Obesity*, ed. John Cawley (New York: Oxford University Press, 2011), 36–37.

80 Abigail Saguy, *What's Wrong with Fat?* (New York: Oxford University Press, 2013), 8.

81 Harvard T. H. Chan School of Public Health, "An Epidemic of Obesity: U.S. Obesity Trends," *The Nutrition Source*, http://www.hsph.harvard.edu/nutritionsource/an-epidemic-of-obesity.

82 This survey, conducted through the ProQuest digital archive of historical newspapers, was restricted to a 1990–2015 date range and U.S. publication.

83 The epidemic metaphor works both ways and some diet leaders upend the disease metaphor by calling for a "health addiction." In his 2005 *Quit Digging Your Grave with a Knife and Fork,* former Arkansas governor Mike Huckabee described his "hope and goal" that healthy behavior "will spread like a highly contagious but benevolent virus." Gordon Mitchell and Kathleen McTigue, "The US Obesity 'Epidemic': Metaphor, Method, or Madness?," *Social Epistemology* 21, no. 4 (October–December 2007): 415; Mike Huckabee, *Quit Digging Your Grave with a Knife and Fork: A 12-Stop Program to End Bad Habits and Begin a Healthy Lifestyle* (New York: Center Street, 2005), 155.

84 Katharina Vester, *A Taste of Power: Food and American Identities* (Berkeley: University of California Press, 2015), 8.

1   PALEOLITHIC DIETS AND THE CAVEMAN UTOPIA

1 Elizabeth Somer, *The Origin Diet: How Eating Like Our Stone Age Ancestors Will Maximize Your Health* (New York: Henry Holt, 2001), 9–10.

2 Chris Kresser, *Your Personal Paleo Code: The 3-Step Plan to Lose Weight, Reverse Disease, and Stay Fit and Healthy for Life* (New York: Little, Brown, 2013).

3 Diana Rodgers, "Eating Paleo Can Save the World," *Robb Wolf: Revolutionary Solutions to Modern Life* (blog), January 13, 2013, https://robbwolf.com/2016/01/13/eating-paleo-can-save-the-world/.

4 Mark Sisson, correspondence to author, March 2014.

5 Though diets often borrow scientific terminology such as Neanderthals, Cro-Magnons, or troglodytes, most use the term "caveman" to evoke cultural meaning rather than scientific taxonomy. This book uses "caveman" to draw upon this constellation of cultural meanings and "Paleo" in reference to specifically "Paleo" books published in the wake of Cordain's 2002 *The Paleo Diet.*

6 Tyler Graham, "The Paleo Diet and the Case for Primal Living," *Men's Journal*, December 2012, http://www.mensjournal.com/magazine/the-paleo-diet-and-the-case-for-primal -living-20130226.

7 Chris Kresser, *Personal Paleo Code* (New York: Little, Brown, 2013), 20.

8 Seth Roberts, qtd. in John Durant, *The Paleo Manifesto: Ancient Wisdom for Lifelong Health* (New York: Random House, 2013), back cover.

9 Durant, *Paleo Manifesto*, 13.

10 Ruth Levitas, *The Concept of Utopia* (London: Philip Allan, 1990), 141.

11 Fedon Lindberg, *The GI Mediterranean Diet* (Berkeley, CA: Ulysses Press, 2009), 92; Robb Wolf, *The Paleo Solution: The Original Human Diet* (Las Vegas, NV: Victory Belt, 2010), 30; Valerie Alston, *Paleo Smoothies* (n.p.: Mihails Konoplovs, 2014), 1.

12 S. Boyd Eaton, Marjorie Shostak, and Melvin Konner, *The Paleolithic Prescription: A Program of Diet & Exercise and a Design for Living* (New York: Harper & Row, 1988), 1.

13 Wolf, *Paleo Solution*, 40.

14 John Warner, *Rousseau and the Problem of Human Relations* (University Park: Pennsylvania State University Press, 2015), 66.

15 Ibid., iii, 50. By the time of his diet activism, Densmore and his brothers had already invented the tanked railroad oil car and funded the first typewriter. "Densmore typewriters" are responsible for the QWERTY letter pattern still used today. When he died in 1911, Densmore bequeathed much of his fortune to the Tuskegee Institute, the historically black university founded by Booker T. Washington. Densmore left the university more than $750,000, or around $18 million in today's dollars (The Month's Review: What Educational People Are Doing and Saying," *The American Educational Review*, 33, no.4 [January 1912]: 165).

16 Gregory, James, *Of Victorians and Vegetarians: The Vegetarian Movement in Nineteenth-Century Britain* (London: Tauris Academic Studies, 2007), 80.

17 John Harvey Kellogg, *The Natural Diet of Man* (Battle Creek, MI: Modern Medicine Publishing Company, 1923), 29.

18 The terminology can be misleading because the nuances of "caveman" have changed over time. The 1920s burst of caveman-themed nutritional advice appears more dramatic in the media coverage than the primary sources would indicate, because "caveman" was more often used as shorthand for meat-heavy or low-carbohydrate diets in the first half of the twentieth century. Reporters sometimes editorialized, calling diet plans "caveman diets" even when their original authors did not use the term.

19 "Lauds Caveman's Diet," *The Chicago Defender*, March 27, 1926.

20 "Holds Missionaries Degrade Pagan Races," *The New York Times*, February 20, 1926.

21 Walter Voegtlin, *The Stone Age Diet: Based on In-Depth Studies of Human Ecology and the Diet of Man* (New York: Vantage Press, 1975), 12, 260.

22 Herman Taller's 1961 *Calories Don't Count* also advocated for a low-carbohydrate diet, but the scandal following his indictment on counts of drug violations, postal fraud, and conspiracy tainted his image and the low-carbohydrate approach. After the FDA found Taller guilty of huckstering his "worthless" safflower oil pills, FDA commissioner George Larrick issued a statement in 1962 declaring that, contrary to Taller's claims,

"calories do count." This high-profile case resulted in the seizure of over a million copies of the paperback and provided damning evidence against low-carbohydrate plans.

23 Leslie Womble and Thomas Wadden, "Commercial and Self-Help Weight Loss Programs," in *Eating Disorders and Obesity: A Comprehensive Handbook*, ed. Christopher G. Fairburn and Kelly D. Brownell (New York: Guilford Press, 2002), 546–550.

24 Voegtlin, *The Stone Age Diet*, 13.

25 Constance Areson Clark, "Evolution for John Doe: Pictures, the Public, and the Scopes Trial Debate," *Journal of American History* 87 (2001): 1275–1303.

26 Constance Areson Clark, *God—or Gorilla: Images of Evolution in the Jazz Age* (Baltimore: Johns Hopkins University Press, 2008), 13.

27 Peter Stearns, *Fat History: Bodies and Beauty in the Modern West* (New York: New York University Press, 1997), 3.

28 Joan Jacobs Brumberg, *The Body Project: An Intimate History of American Girls* (New York: Random House, 1997), 99–100.

29 Michael Kimmel, *The History of Men: Essays in the History of American and British Masculinities* (New York: State University of New York Press, 2005), 82.

30 Deborah Levine, "Corpulence and Correspondence: President William H. Taft and the Medical Management of Obesity," *Annals of Internal Medicine* 159, no. 8 (2013): 565–570.

31 Sharlene Hesse-Biber, *The Cult of Thinness* (New York: Oxford University Press, 2007), 42.

32 Susan Bordo, "Hunger as Ideology," in *Eating Culture*, ed. Ron Scapp and Brian Seitz (Albany: State University of New York Press, 1998), 13.

33 Lewis, *The American Adam*, 5.

34 Voegtlin, *The Stone Age Diet*, 253.

35 Ibid., 249–256.

36 S. Boyd Eaton and Melvin Konner, "Paleolithic Nutrition—A Consideration of Its Nature and Current Implications," *New England Journal of Medicine* 312 (January 31, 1985): 283–289.

37 "Affluenza," or the psychological cost of affluence, is the psychological equivalent of these physical diseases of civilization.

38 Eaton and Konner, "Paleolithic Nutrition," 283.

39 For an excellent summary of the scholarly consensus refuting (or at least debating) Eaton and Konner's claims, please see evolutionary biologist Marlene Zuk, *Paleofantasy: What Evolution Really Tells Us about Sex, Diet, and How We Live* (New York: W. W. Norton, 2013). Zuk's discussion of "experimental evolution" is particularly pertinent to arguments discrediting the "stalling" or "peaking" of evolutionary processes in the Paleolithic (67–92).

40 Eaton and Konner, "Paleolithic Nutrition," 284. This figure was later corrected in the April issue of the *New England Journal of Medicine*. The editors amended the "six inches" to "12.2 cm (4.8 inches)" but the correction was largely unnoticed and most Paleo books still neglect the April 1985 correction.

41 Douglas Crews and Barry Bogin, "Growth, Development, Senescence, and Aging: A Life History Perspective," in *A Companion to Biological Anthropology*, ed. Clark Spencer Larsen (Oxford: Wiley-Blackwell, 2010), 139–144.

42 Loren Cordain, *The Real Paleo Diet Cookbook* (New York: Houghton Mifflin Harcourt, 2015), 13.

43 Loren Cordain, *The Paleo Answer: 7 Days to Lose Weight, Feel Great, Stay Young* (Hoboken, NJ: John Wiley & Sons, 2010), 3.

44 Mark Sisson, "About," *Mark's Daily Apple,* http://www.marksdailyapple.com/about-2/mark-sisson/#axzz3DFQectPn; Mark Sisson, correspondence to author, March 2014. For a curated list of the top 100 blogs (from well over a thousand), see Joel Runyon, "100+ Incredible Paleo Diet Blogs," *Ultimate Paleo Guide,* http://ultimatepaleoguide.com/paleo-diet-blogs/.

45 The Ancestral Health Society, "Manifesto," *About AHS,* http://www.ancestralhealth.org/about.

46 Jacque Wilson, "Paleo Diet Ranks Last on 'Best Diets' List," *CNN,* January 7, 2014, http://www.cnn.com/2014/01/07/health/best-diets-ranked/.

47 Lyman Tower Sargent, *Utopianism: A Very Short Introduction* (Oxford: Oxford University Press, 2010), 127.

48 Ibid.

49 Ibid.

50 Lewis, *The American Adam,* 9.

51 Friedrich Nietzsche, *The Use and Abuse of History,* trans. Adrian Collins (Indianapolis, IN: Bobbs-Merrill, 1957), 5–6.

52 Lewis, *The American Adam,* 5.

53 F. O. Matthiessen, qtd. in Shelley Fisher Fishkin, *From Fact to Fiction: Journalism and Imaginative Writing in America* (New York: Oxford University Press, 1985), 5.

54 Somer, *Origin Diet,* 195, xvi.

55 Louis Marin, *Food for Thought* (Baltimore: Johns Hopkins University Press, 1989), 107.

56 Levitas, *Concept of Utopia,* 3.

57 Mikhail Bakhtin, *Rabelais and His World* (Cambridge, MA: MIT Press, 1968), 170–171.

58 Amy Bingaman, Lise Sanders, and Rebecca Zorach, *Embodied Utopias: Gender, Social Change, and the Modern Metropolis* (London: Routledge, 2002), 2.

59 S. Boyd Eaton, Melvin Konner, and Marjorie Shostak, "Stone Agers in the Fast Lane: Chronic Degenerative Diseases in Evolutionary Perspective," *The American Journal of Medicine* 84, no. 4 (1988): 739–749; Eaton et al., *The Paleolithic Prescription.*

60 See Susie Orbach, *Fat Is a Feminist Issue: The Anti-Diet Guide to Permanent Weight Loss* (New York: Paddington Press, 1978); Jana Evans Braziel and Kathleen LeBesco, eds., *Bodies out of Bounds: Fatness and Transgression* (Berkeley: University of California Press, 2001).

61 David Schwartz and Hamilton Stapell, "Modern Cavemen? Stereotypes and Reality of the Ancestral Health Movement," *Journal of Evolution and Health* 1, no. 1 (2013): 2–10.

62 Katharina Vester, *A Taste of Power: Food and American Identities* (Berkeley: University of California Press, 2015), 12.

63 Nell Stephenson, *Paleoista: Gain Energy, Get Lean and Feel Fabulous with the Diet You Were Born to Eat* (New York: Simon & Schuster, 2012), 4.

64 Hugh Campbell, Michael Bell, and Margaret Finney, *Country Boys: Masculinity and Rural Life* (University Park: Pennsylvania State University Press, 2006), 159.

65 Susan Bordo, *Unbearable Weight: Feminism, Western Culture, and the Body* (Berkeley: University of California Press, 2003), 130.

66 "Gender Bias" (online forum post), *Paleo Hacks Cave*, May 21, 2012, http://paleo hacks.com/paleo/is-there-a-gender-bias-inherent-in-a-meat-heavy-paleo-diet-16107.

67 Summer Innanen, "Breaking the Diet-Sabotage Cycle," poster and program at the Ancestral Health Society Symposium, Berkeley, CA, August 2014.

68 Claire Yates, *Optimum Health the Paleo Way* (Wollombi, NSW, Australia: Exisle Publishing, 2013), 5; Joseph Salama and Christina Lianos, eds., *The Paleo Miracle* (n.p.: The Paleo Miracle, LLC, 2012), 153.

69 See Shari Dworkin and Faye Wachs's study of the historical shift towards the "fit ideal" in their *Body Panic: Gender, Health, and the Selling of Fitness* (New York: New York University Press, 2009).

70 Esther Blum, *Cavewomen Don't Get Fat* (New York: Gallery Books, 2013), 20.

71 Arthur de Vany, *The New Evolution Diet: What Our Paleolithic Ancestors Can Teach Us about Weight Loss, Fitness, and Aging* (Emmaus, PA: Rodale Press, 2010), 2.

72 Jani Zubkovs, *Why Women Love Cavemen—A Man's Guide to Tame the Bitch* (New York: Bonnie's Gang, 2009).

73 David Clarke, *Cinderella Meets the Caveman* (Eugene, OR: Harvest House Publishers, 2007), 114, 97.

74 Martha McCaughey, *The Caveman Mystique: Pop-Darwinism and the Debates over Sex, Violence, and Science* (New York: Routledge, 2008), 12–14.

75 John Pettegrew, *Brutes in Suits: Male Sensibility in America, 1890–1920* (Baltimore: Johns Hopkins University Press, 2007), 321.

76 Pierre Bourdieu, *Masculine Domination* (Stanford, CA: Stanford University Press, 2001), 23. Emphasis in original.

77 Eaton et al., *Paleolithic Prescription*, 260–261.

78 Ibid., 263–264.

79 Loren Cordain, *The Paleo Diet* (Hoboken, NJ: John Wiley & Sons, 2002), 135.

80 Wolf, *Paleo Solution*, 33.

81 Dana Carpender, *500 Paleo Recipes: Hundreds of Delicious Recipes for Weight Loss and Super Health* (Beverly, MA: Fair Winds Press, 2012), 13. Emphasis in original.

82 Jean Hofve and Celeste Yarnall, *Paleo Dog: Give Your Best Friend a Long Life, Healthy Weight, and Freedom from Illness by Nurturing His Inner Wolf* (Emmaus, PA: Rodale Press, 2014), 143.

83 Darko Suvin, *Metamorphoses of Science Fiction: On the Poetics and History of a Literary Genre* (New Haven, CT: Yale University Press, 1979), 49.

84 Tatiana Teslenko, *Feminist Utopian Novels of the 1970s: Joanna Russ & Dorothy Bryant* (New York: Routledge, 2003), 28.

85 Eaton et al., *Paleolithic Prescription*, 24.

86 Loren Cordain, *The Paleo Diet for Athletes* (Emmaus, PA: Rodale Press, 2005), xv; Alissa Friedman, interview by author, Berkeley, CA, August 2014.

87 Grace Kim, interview by author, Stanford, CA, January 2013.

88 Ruth Levitas, "Educated Hope: Ernst Bloch on Abstract and Concrete Utopia," *Utopian Studies* 1, no. 2 (1990): 18.

89 Ibid., 14–18.

90 Victoria Pitts, *In the Flesh: The Cultural Politics of Body Modification* (New York: Palgrave Macmillan, 2003), 31.

91 Anthony Giddens, *Modernity and Self-Identity: Self and Society in the Late Modern Age* (Stanford, CA: Stanford University Press, 1991), 281.

92 Meg Cannon, "Women of Crossfit = Strong" (post), *Facebook*, September 4, 2014, https://www.facebook.com/CFStrongWomen/.

93 "Our Mission," *Paleo Foundation*, March 11, 2014, http://paleofoundation.org/about-us/.

94 Ibid.

95 "Mission," *Wild Man Foods*, http://www.wildmanfoods.org/mission.

96 Blum, *Cavewomen Don't Get Fat*, 114.

97 Melissa Joulwan and Kellyann Petrucci, *Living Paleo for Dummies* (Hoboken, NJ: John Wiley & Sons, 2013), iii.

98 Somer, *Origin Diet*, dedication.

99 Friedman, interview, 2014; Pauli Halstead, Primal Cuisine (Rochester, VT: Healing Arts Press, 2012), 19.

100 Jane Barthelemy, *Paleo Desserts* (Boston: Da Capo Press, 2012), 5.

101 See Henning Steinfeld, *Livestock's Long Shadow—Environmental Issues and Options* (Rome: Food and Agriculture Organization of the United Nations, 2006), for a comprehensive and well-received assessment of the environmental costs of meat.

102 James Kopp, "Cosimo Noto's The Ideal City (1903): New Orleans as Medical Utopia," *Utopian Studies* 1, no. 2 (1990): 115–122.

103 Others define the period more generously, including the Upper and Lower Paleolithic eras; for example, Joulwan and Petrucci in *Living Paleo for Dummies* define their diet by the 2.49-million-year period when they write that "early man was called a *hunter-gatherer*" (10).

104 Bob Smeja, "Adam and Eve," *Paleo by God's Design* (blog), July 10, 2012, http://designerpaleo.blogspot.com.es/2012/07/.

105 Roy Mankovitz, *The Original Diet: The Omnivore's Solution Designed by Nature, Researched by a Rocket Scientist* (Santa Barbara, CA: Montecito Wellness, 2008), 8.

106 Eaton et al., *Paleolithic Prescription*, 3.

107 Ibid.

108 Ibid.

109 Mark Sisson, *The Primal Connection: Follow Your Genetic Blueprint to Health and Happiness* (Malibu, CA: Primal Nutrition, 2013), 66.

110 Of Sargent's eight characteristics of mythic Eutopias, the paradise described in the caveman diet only violates the feature of "no enmity between homo sapiens and the other animals." Not only do cavemen regularly hunt (usually big animals with spears or arrows) but animals are also described as similarly terrorizing cavemen prey in the "eat or get eaten!" predacious world. Lyman Tower Sargent, "The Three Faces of Utopianism Revisited," *Utopian Studies* 5, no. 1 (1994): 10; Mark Sisson, *The Primal Blueprint: Reprogram Your Genes for Effortless Weight Loss, Vibrant Health, and Boundless Energy* (Malibu, CA: Primal Nutrition, 2012), 14.

111 Brenda Garrett, "England, Colonialism, and 'The Land of Cokaygne,'" *Utopian Studies* 15, no. 1 (2004): 1–12; M. Usman and John Davidson, *Paleo Diet—Good or Bad?* (Mendon, UT: JD-Biz Publishing, Health Learning Series, 2013).

112 Sargent, "Three Faces of Utopianism Revisited," 10.

113 Kate Fredericks, *What Is Paleo Diet?* (n.p.: CreateSpace Independent Publishing Platform eBook, 2012), 18.

114 Darryl Edwards, with Brett Stewart and Jason Warner, *Paleo Fitness* (Berkeley, CA: Ulysses Press, 2013), 41.

115 Somer, *Origin Diet*, 9.

116 Ibid., 10–11.

117 Jeanne Floresca, *Paleo Traveler: Old World Recipes Flipped NeoPaleo* (n.p.: Bookbaby, 2014), 2.

118 Wolf, *Paleo Solution*, 120.

119 Joulwan and Petrucci, *Living Paleo for Dummies*, 12.

120 Kenneth Russ, *The Palm Springs Diet: An Old Stone Age Diet for Modern Times* (Bloomington, IN: AuthorHouse, 2007).

121 Eaton et al., *Paleo Prescription*, 1.

122 Oliver Selway, *Instinctive Fitness* (Herts, AL: Ecademy Press, 2012).

123 Ori Hofmekler and Diana Holtzberg, *The Warrior Diet* (St. Paul, MN: Dragon Door Publications, 2001), xxx.

124 Voegtlin, *The Stone Age Diet*, 161.

125 Ibid., 12.

126 Blum, *Cavewomen Don't Get Fat*, 79.

127 Telamon Press, *The Paleo Weight Loss Plan* (Berkeley, CA: Telamon Press, 2013).

128 Robert S. Fogarty, "An Imaginary Country" (Editorial), *Antioch Review* 63, no. 4 (Autumn 2005): 613–614.

129 Lyman Tower Sargent, *Utopianism: A Very Short Introduction* (Oxford: Oxford University Press, 2010), 12.

130 Garrett, "England, Colonialism, and 'The Land of Cokaygne,'" 2.

131 Ibid.

132 Jennie Harrell, "Is Paleo Expensive?," *EasyPaleo* (blog), January 28, 2012, http://www.easypaleo.com/2012/01/28/is-paleo-expensive-my-thoughts-money-saving-tips/.

133 In the tradition set by that fateful apple, many Christian diets have similarly decried "deceitful foods." A 1976 diet, *More of Jesus, Less of Me*, argues that "cakes and milkshakes won't lose their calories because you pray over them! In addition to being loaded with calories, these sweet gooeyes are 'deceitful foods' because they cause addiction to themselves." Joan Cavanaugh and Pat Forseth, *More of Jesus, Less of Me* (Plainfield, NJ: Logos International, 1976), 96.

134 Sarah Hill, *Paleo Diet* (n.p.: MaxHouse eBook, 2013), 7.

135 Stuart Berger, *Dr. Berger's Immune Power Diet* (New York: New American Library, 1985), 71.

136 Loren Cordain, *The Paleo Diet Cookbook* (Hoboken, NJ: John Wiley & Sons, 2011), 184.

137 Voegtlin, *Stone Age Diet*, 4.

138 Jean-Pierre de Villiers, *77 Ways to Reshape Your Life* (Herts, AL: Ecademy Press, 2011), n.p.

139 Cordain, *Paleo Diet Cookbook*, 184.

140 Cordain, *Paleo Diet*, 127.

141 Ibid.

142 Cordain, *Paleo Diet Cookbook*, 3.

143 Ray Audette, with Troy Gilchrist, *Neanderthin: Eat Like a Caveman to Achieve a Lean, Strong, Healthy Body* (New York: St. Martin's Press, 1999), 71.

144 Jodie Cohen and Gilaad Cohen, *The Everything Paleolithic Diet Book: An All-Natural, Easy-to-Follow Plan to Improve Health, Lose Weight, Increase Endurance, Prevent Disease* (Avon, MA: Adams Media, 2011), 23.

145 Etta Madden and Martha L. Finch, *Eating in Eden: Food and American Utopias* (Lincoln: University of Nebraska Press, 2006), 4.

146 Ibid., 2.

147 Levitas, *Concept of Utopia*, 141.

148 Steven R. Gundry, *Dr. Gundry's Diet Evolution* (New York: Crown Publishers, 2008), 1.

149 Blum, *Cavewomen Don't Get Fat*, 24.

150 Eaton et al., *Paleolithic Prescription*, 132.

151 Joseph Winters, "Toward an Embodied Utopia: Marcuse, the Re-Ordering of Desire, and the 'Broken' Promise of Post-Liberal Practices," *Telos*, no. 165 (Winter 2013): 151–168.

152 James Villepigue and Rick Collins, *Alpha Male Challenge* (Emmaus, PA: Rodale Press, 2009), 91.

153 Anthony Burlay, *The Foundation Diet: Your Body Was Designed to Eat* (W. Hollywood, CA: Zen-Fusion Publishing, 2004), 45.

154 Kim, interview with author, 2013. "Maybe I can" could be interpreted as "Yes we can" written in the vulnerable, tentative language of the self. It isn't an accident that "Yes We Can" and "Make America Great Again" have been defining American presidential campaign slogans. They are two sides of the same coin: the future and the past. Taken together, we see the same unrelenting message so clear in the diet books, looking back to a better past, mourning a fallen present, drafting plans for a more perfect world.

155 Boston Medical Center, "Weight Management," *Nutrition and Weight Management*, http://www.bmc.org/nutritionweight/services/weightmanagement.htm. Adding to the irony, yo-yo dieting (technically, "weight cycling") has been shown to increase the difficulty of warding off weight regain after initial periods of dramatic loss. Put another way, the more one diets, the harder it is to get and stay thin.

156 Durant, *Paleo Manifesto*, 290.

2 DEVOTIONAL DIETS AND THE AMERICAN EDEN

1 George Malkmus, with Peter and Stowe Shockey, *The Hallelujah Diet: Experience the Optimal Health You Were Meant to Have* (Shippensburg, PA: Destiny Image Publishers, 2006), 35.

2 These terms connote subtle differences. "Christian diets" describes texts that refer to specific Christian denominations, authored by ordained clergy, or published by Christian publishing houses such as Personal Christianity or Zondervan. "Devotional diets" such as *Greater Health, God's Way* (1984) describe texts that rely on the rhetoric of godly or holy foods, rather than Jesus himself. "Eden diets" such as *The Eden Diet* (2010) can encompass both devotional and Christian diets, but the term specifically refers to those texts set in Eden and most often modeled after the diet of Adam and Eve.

3 R. Marie Griffith, *Born Again Bodies: Flesh and Spirit in American Christianity* (Berkeley: University of California Press, 2004), 172.

4 "About Jordan Rubin," *The Maker's Diet*, http://makersdiet.com/about.php.

5 Anugrah Kumar, "Rick Warren Leads Church Members to Lose 250,000 Pounds in One Year," *The Christian Post*, January 15, 2012, http://www.christianpost.com/news/-rick-warren-leads-church-members-to-lose-250000-pounds-in-one-year-67200/#yUZ6uLyWMoldlyab.99.

6 Leslie Leyland Fields, "The Fitness-Driven Church," *Christianity Today*, June 21, 2013, http://www.christianitytoday.com/ct/2013/june/fitness-driven-church.html.

7 Joan Cavanaugh and Pat Forseth, *More of Jesus, Less of Me* (Plainfield, NJ: Logos International, 1976); C. S. Lovett, *Help Lord—The Devil Wants Me Fat!* (Baldwin Park, CA: Personal Christianity, 1977); Stormie Omartian, *Greater Health, God's Way: Seven Steps to Health, Youthfulness and Vitality* (Canoga Park, CA: Sparrow Press, 1984); Jennifer Garth, *Adam and Eve Weren't Fat* (Milsons Point, NSW: Random House Australia, 1999); Shannon Tanner, *Diets Don't Work . . . But Jesus Does!* (Maitland, FL: Xulon Press, 2007); Rachel Albert-Matesz and Don Matesz, *The Garden of Eating: A Produce-Dominated Diet & Cookbook* (Phoenix, AZ: Planetary Press, 2004); Antonio Costantini, H. Wieland, and Lars I. Qvick, *The Garden of Eden Longevity Diet: Antifungal-Antimycotoxin Diet for the Prevention and Treatment of Cancer, Atherosclerosis (Coronary-Carotid Vascular Disease) and Other Degenerative Diseases* (Freiburg, Germany: Oberlin, 1998); Charles H. Wharton, *Metabolic Man: Ten Thousand Years from Eden: The Long Search for a Personal Nutrition from Our Forest Origins to the Supermarkets of Today* (Orlando, FL: Winmark Publishing, 2001); Rita Hancock, *The Eden Diet: You Can Eat Treats, Enjoy Your Food, and Lose Weight* (Grand Rapids, MI: Zondervan, 2010).

8 Religiosity alone does not explain the obesity rate disparity: religious Christians are much more likely to be obese than members of other religious denominations and, perhaps, this disparity might account for the dearth of Jewish, Muslim, or other religious diets. However, research suggests that Christian diets are more firmly rooted in the narrative of the Fall of Man, more direct inheritors of the American jeremiad tradition, and more invested in the Edenic vision of a healthy, pure landscape. Likewise, the laws of Kashrut and Halal already characterize Judaism and Islam, respectively, and

a specific Jewish or Muslim commercial weight loss diet might be inimical to those dietary laws.

9 Christopher Ellison and Jeffrey Levin, "The Religion-Health Connection: Evidence, Theory, and Future Directions," *Health Education and Behavior* 25, no. 6 (1998): 700–720.

10 Though most studies of the religion-health connection have examined mental health, gerontological research has shown religious attendance linked to better measures of morbidity and mortality. Other studies connect religious involvement with reduced rates of heart disease, stroke, and gastrointestinal disease. Since most religious people live longer, healthier lives than the general population, increased obesity prevalence in religious Christians is a puzzling outlier.

11 Dana Cassell and David Gleaves, "Religion and Obesity," in *The Encyclopedia of Obesity and Eating Disorders* (New York: Infobase Publishing, 2006), 258. Diet leader La Vita Weaver confirms the theory, writing that "food has taken the place of those other desires" fulfilled by "getting drunk, using drugs, or having sex." La Vita Weaver, *Fit for God: The 8-Week Plan That Kicks the Devil Out and Invites Health and Healing In* (New York: Doubleday, 2004), 183.

12 K. H. Kim, J. Sobal, and E. Wethington, "Religion and Body Weight," *International Journal of Obesity and Related Metabolic Disorders* 27, no. 4 (April 2003): 469–477.

13 Alexandra Wolfe, "Pastor Rick Warren: Fighting Obesity with Faith," *The Wall Street Journal*, January 17, 2014.

14 Peter Stearns, *Fat History: Bodies and Beauty in the Modern West* (New York: New York University Press, 1997), 208.

15 Harvey Levenstein, *Fear of Food: A History of Why We Worry about What We Eat* (Chicago: University of Chicago Press, 2012), 3–4.

16 Elizabeth Sharon Hayenga, "Dieting through the Decades: A Comparative Study of Weight Reduction in America as Depicted in Popular Literature and Books from 1940 to the Late 1980s" (PhD diss., University of Minnesota, 1989), 12.

17 Joan Jacobs Brumberg, "Fasting Girls: The Emerging Ideal of Slenderness in American Culture," in *Women's America: Refocusing the Past*, 8th ed., ed. Linda Kerber, Jane Sherron de Hart, Cornelia Hughes Dayton, and Judy Tzu-Chun Wu (New York: Oxford University Press, 2016), 422.

18 Michelle Lelwica, "Fulfilling Femininity and Transcending the Flesh: Traditional Religious Beliefs and Gender Ideals in Popular Women's Magazines," *Online Journal of Religion and Society* 1 (1999), 9.

19 Paul Campos, *The Obesity Myth: Why America's Obsession with Weight Is Hazardous to Your Health* (New York: Gotham Books, 2004), xxi.

20 See also Caroline Walker Bynum, *Holy Feast and Holy Fast: The Religious Significance of Food to Medieval Women* (Berkeley: University of California Press, 1987) for medieval Christian traditions of food refusal, femininity, and asceticism.

21 Joan Jacobs Brumberg, *Fasting Girls: The Emergence of Anorexia Nervosa as a Modern Disease* (Cambridge, MA: Harvard University Press, 1988); Amanda Porterfield, *Female Piety in Puritan New England: The Emergence of Religious Humanism* (New York: Oxford University Press, 1992).

22 Brumberg also distinguishes modern "anorexia" from older forms of fasting to argue that, though self-discipline characterized both forms, contemporary anorexia emphasizes the willpower of the individual over the saintliness of the fasting saint's religious calling.

23 Porterfield, *Female Piety in Puritan New England*, 126.

24 Ibid.

25 Lelwica, "Fulfilling Femininity and Transcending the Flesh," 8; William James Hoverd, *Working Out My Salvation: The Contemporary Gym and the Promise of "Self" Transformation* (Oxford: Meyer & Meyer Sport, 2005), 30–34.

26 Griffith, *Born Again Bodies*, 12.

27 Samantha Kwan and Christine Soriea Sheikh, "Divine Dieting: A Cultural Analysis of Christian Weight Loss Programs," in *Food and Faith: Eating in the Christian Tradition*, ed. Kenneth Albala and Trudy Eden (New York: Columbia University Press, 2011), 215.

28 Robert M. Schwartz, *Holy Eating: The Spiritual Secret to Eternal Weight Loss* (Bloomington, IN: iUniverse, 2012), 8; Hancock, *The Eden Diet*, 112.

29 Laura Harris Smith, *The 30-Day Faith Detox: Renew Your Mind, Cleanse Your Body, Heal Your Spirit* (Bloomington, MN: Chosen Books, 2016), 52.

30 Hancock, *The Eden Diet*, 111–112.

31 Marie Chapian and Neva Coyle, *Free to Be Thin* (Minneapolis, MN: Bethany House, 1979), 64.

32 R. Marie Griffith, "'Don't Eat That': The Erotics of Abstinence in American Christianity," *Gastronomica: The Journal of Food and Culture* 1, no. 4 (Fall 2001): 43.

33 Bruce T. Marshall, "The Theology of Eating," *Christian Century* 98 (March 18, 1981): 301–302.

34 Rachel Marie Stone, *Eat with Joy: Redeeming God's Gift of Food* (Downers Grove, IL: InterVarsity Press, 2013), 24.

35 Lynne Gerber, "Fat Christians and Fit Elites: Negotiating Class and Status in Evangelical Christian Weight-Loss Culture," *American Quarterly* 64, no. 1 (March 2012): 63.

36 Charles Shedd, *Pray Your Weight Away* (Philadelphia: Lippincott, 1957), 15.

37 Deborah Pierce, as told to Frances Spatz Leighton, "I Prayed Myself Slim," *The Washington Post*, April 10, 1960.

38 Griffith, *Born Again Bodies*, 172.

39 Ibid.

40 J. Dart, "Book Pits Faith against Fat," *Los Angeles Times*, July 10, 1976.

41 John Kennedy, "The Weigh Down Heresy," *Journal of the Southern Baptist Convention* (November 2000), www.sbclife.net/articles/2000/11/sla7.

42 Griffith, *Born Again Bodies*, 172.

43 Victoria Pitts, *In the Flesh: The Cultural Politics of Body Modification* (New York: Palgrave Macmillan, 2003), 31.

44 A minority of these diets published in the last twenty years still hold the obese directly liable for their condition and discredit the environment or state of the nation. For example, Elvin Adams writes plainly in 2011 that "this book is aimed at the defect in you that prevents diets from working." Still, however, Adams blames "genes" more broadly because, as he writes, "Eve lost control over herself. . . . The indulgence of appetite is in your defective genes. This defect has been passed down over all the generations and is growing worse today." Elvin Adams, *Jesus Was Thin So You Can Be Thin Too* (Blooming-ton, IN: iUniverse, 2011), xi, 19.

45 Charlie Shedd, *The Fat Is in Your Head* (New York: Avon Books, 1972), 13.

46 Ibid., 62.

47 Centers for Disease Control and Prevention, "Adult Obesity Facts," *Overweight and Obesity*, September 9, 2014, http://www.cdc.gov/obesity/data/adult.html.

48 Malkmus, *The Hallelujah Diet*, 144.

49 Gene Wall Cole, *Jesus' Diet for All the World* (Henrietta, NC: A.I. Publishing, 2005), ix.

50 Kara Davis, *Spiritual Secrets to Weight Loss* (Lake Mary, FL: Charisma Media, 2002), 70, 90.

51 Rick Warren, Daniel Amen, and Mark Hyman, *The Daniel Plan: 40 Days to a Health-ier Life* (Grand Rapids, MI: Zondervan, 2013), 8.

52 Ted Haggard, *The Jerusalem Diet: The "One Day" Approach to Reach Your Ideal Weight—and Stay There* (Colorado Springs, CO: Waterbrook Press, 2005), 2.

53 Weaver, *Fit for God*, 198–199.

54 Kwan and Sheikh, "Divine Dieting," 215–216.

55 Donald Miller, *Easy Health Diet: Manage Weight and Prevent Scary Diseases* (Salt Lake City, UT: Thimk.Biz, 2004), 143

56 Weaver, *Fit for God*, 204.

57 Edward Dumke, *The Serpent Beguiled Me and I Ate: A Heavenly Diet for Saints and Sinners* (Garden City, NY: Doubleday, 1986), 5.

58 I chose Malkmus, Hancock, and Rubin not only for the richness of their texts but for the diversity of their backgrounds. Hancock is a board-certified medical doctor. Conversely, Malkmus does not claim official medical expertise, and even his ordination as a reverend is dubious. Malkmus never attended divinity school or seminary and has never professed allegiance to any particular denomination. Malkmus may have enrolled in a free online ordination program, so he might technically be certified but, still, his credentials are suspect. Rubin's credentials are of hazy provenance. His NMD (naturo-pathic medical doctor), PhD, and CNC (certified nutritional consultant) credentials were awarded by nonaccredited correspondence schools that most often grant degrees for a fee.

59 Trust for America's Health and Robert Wood Johnson Foundation, *F as in Fat: How Obesity Threatens America's Future*, August 2013, http://stateofobesity.org/-files/fasin fat2013.pdf.

60 Richard Carmona, "The Obesity Crisis in America," Testimony before the Sub-committee on Educational Reform, Committee on Education and the Workforce, U.S. House of Representatives, July 16, 2003, http://www.surgeongeneral.gov/news/testi mony/obesity07162003.html.

61 Jordan Rubin, *The Maker's Diet Revolution: The 10 Day Diet to Lose Weight and Detox-ify Your Body, Mind and Spirit* (Shippensburg, PA: Destiny Image Publishers, 2013), 33.

62 Stephen Barrett, "Rev. George M. Malkmus and His Hallelujah Diet," *Quackwatch*, May 29, 2013, http://www.quackwatch.org/11Ind/-malkmus.html.

63 George Malkmus, interview with Donna Sundblad, "Hallelujah Diet Founder George Malkmus," *Lovetoknow*, http://diet.lovetoknow-.com/wiki/Hallelujah_Diet_Founder _George_Malkmus.

64 Martha Quillin, "Eats of Eden," *McClatchy-Tribune Business News*, December 10, 2006, 1.

65 Malkmus, *The Hallelujah Diet*, 57.

66 Ibid., 46.

67 Ibid., 45.

68 Ibid.

69 Ibid., 32–45.

70 Ibid., 39.

71 When pressed about the actual effects of the supplement, a Hallelujah Diet sales representative explained that the Get Started Kit ($59.95) will "detox" the body, most likely causing "headache, fatigue, and flu-like symptoms" for a week.

72 Malkmus, *The Hallelujah Diet*, 94.

73 Ibid., 218.

74 Ibid., 79.

75 Ibid., 37, 58.

76 Jordan Rubin, *The Maker's Diet: The 40-Day Health Experience That Will Change Your Life Forever* (Shippensburg, PA: Destiny Image Publishers, 2004), 3, 30.

77 "About Jordan Rubin," *The Maker's Diet*, http://makersdiet.com/about.php.

78 Jordan Rubin, *Patient Heal Thyself: A Remarkable Health Program Combining Ancient Wisdom with Groundbreaking Clinical Research* (Topanga, CA: Freedom Press, 2003).

79 Federal Trade Commission, "Dietary Supplement Maker Garden of Life Settles FTC Charges" (press release), March 9, 2006, https://www.ftc.gov/news-events/press -releases/2006/03/dietary-supplement-maker-garden-life-settles-ftc-charges.

80 Ibid.

81 Jordan Rubin, *The Maker's Diet: The 40-Day Health Experience*, 2.

82 Ibid.

83 Ibid., 32.

84 Jordan Rubin, *The Maker's Diet for Weight Loss: 16-Week Strategy for Burning Fat, Cleansing Toxins, and Living a Healthier Life!* (Lake Mary, FL: Siolam Strang Company, 2009), 15.

85 Rubin, *The Maker's Diet: The 40-Day Health Experience*, 3.

86 Ibid., 49.

87 Ibid., 32–42.

88 Ibid., 43.

89 Ibid., 46.

90 For a masterful analysis of time and Thomas Cole's *Expulsion from the Garden of Eden*, see Bryan Wolf's *Romantic Re-Vision: Culture and Consciousness in Nineteenth-Century American Painting and Literature* (Chicago: University of Chicago Press, 1982).

91 Charles Francis Horne and Julius August Brewer, *The Bible and Its Story: Taught by One Thousand Picture Lessons* (New York: F. R. Niglutsch, 1908), 18.

92 Rick Warren, qtd. in Kris Patrick, "Pastor Rick Warren Hopes to Create New Diet Craze 'The Daniel Plan,'" *Path MEGAzine*, January 8, 2014, http://pathmegazine.com /news/world-news/pastor-rick-warren-hopes-to-create-new-diet-craze-the-daniel-plan/.

93 Perry Miller, *The New England Mind: From Colony to Province* (Cambridge, MA: Harvard University Press, 1953).

94 Sacvan Bercovitch, *The American Jeremiad* (Madison: University of Wisconsin Press, 1978), 176.

95 Ibid., 180.

96 Rubin, *The Maker's Diet*, 2.

97 Stone, *Eat with Joy*, 48.

98 Warren et al., *The Daniel Plan*, 77.

99 Rubin, *The Maker's Diet*, 38.

100 Arthur Halliday and Judy Wardell Halliday, *Get Thin, Stay Thin: A Biblical Approach to Food, Eating, and Weight Management* (Grand Rapids, MI: Revell Books, 2007), 78.

101 James Creed, Jr., *Answers: As the Lightning Cometh out of the East, and Shineth Even unto the West: So Shall Also the Coming of the Son of Man Be* (Bloomington, IN: Xlibris, 2003), 306.

102 Joyce Meyer, *Look Great, Feel Great: 12 Keys to Enjoying a Healthy Life Now* (New York: Warner Faith, 2006), 59.

103 Rubin, *The Maker's Diet*, 39.

104 This argument is similar to Walter Voegtlin's claim in the 1975 *Stone Age Diet* that hunger is a purely "physiological mechanism" but appetite is an "acquired social endowment, a *conditioned* reflex." Voegtlin and his colleagues explained that caveman diets bypass the construct of appetite so the dieter can recognize hunger and, once again, eat intuitively. Walter Voegtlin, *The Stone Age Diet: Based on In-Depth Studies of Human Ecology and the Diet of Man* (New York: Vantage Press, 1975), 161.

105 Stone, *Eat with Joy*, 25.

106 Pam Warmerdam, *The Diet of Eden: How the Low-Carbohydrate Diets Almost Had It Right* (Bloomington, IN: Xlibris, 2011).

107 Weaver, *Fit for God*, 192.

108 Malkmus, *The Hallelujah Diet*, 50.

109 Ibid., 49.

110 Marie Chapian and Neva Coyle, *The All-New Free to Be Thin* (Minneapolis, MN: Bethany House, 1994), 140–163.

111 Adrienna Diona Turner, *The Day Begins with Christ* (n.p.: AuthorHouse, 2009), 89.

112 Stowe Shockey, "Back to the Garden," in Malkmus, *The Hallelujah Diet*, 27–33.

113 Ibid.

114 The theological question of whether you can eat in heaven has raised similar questions about pleasure and godliness. Most of these authors assume that eating is a feature of the afterlife, even though the mortal body does not age or follow any biological clock. In *Life after Death & Heaven and Hell*, the Christian author Brian McAnnaly assures readers that, in heaven, "food and drink [will be] enjoyed in the company of God and other people." He explains, "Eating will not be a necessity in heaven because the eternal bodies that God provides are incorruptible," but people will still eat because "God determined that food is good and pleasing." Brian McAnnaly, *Life after Death & Heaven and Hell* (Capetown, South Africa: Struik Christian Books, 2009), 31.

115 Haggard, *The Jerusalem Diet*, 4.

116 Hancock, *The Eden Diet*, 112.

117 Stone, *Eat with Joy*, 24.

118 Ibid., 32–37.

119 Since the nineteenth century, American landscapes have healed the many ills wrought by modernity; spas, the water cure, even dude ranches all assured greater health through better landscape. The discredited nineteenth-century American theory of medical topography explains the long-standing therapeutic promise of Edenic landscapes. As environmental historian Linda Nash describes it, medical topography theorized that health or disease could be determined by certain qualities of landscape. She clarifies: "For 19th century Americans, bodies themselves were barometers of place" and a region's salubriousness could be judged by its health-giving properties. Linda Nash, "Finishing Nature: Harmonizing Bodies and Environments in Late-Nineteenth-Century California," *Environmental History* 8, no. 1 (January 2003): 26.

120 Malkmus, *The Hallelujah Diet*, 50.

121 Tanner, *Diets Don't Work*, 30–35.

122 Ibid., 32.

123 Lysa TerKeurst, *Made to Crave: Satisfying Your Deepest Desire with God, Not Food* (Grand Rapids, MI: Zondervan, 2011), 22.

124 Tanner, *Diets Don't Work*, 33.

125 Judy Gatehouse, "Home," *Hungry for Jesus*, http://www.hungryforjesus.org.

126 Gwen Shamblin, *The Weigh Down Diet: Gwen Shamblin's Inspirational Way to Lose Weight, Stay Slim, and Find a New You* (New York: Doubleday, 1997), 68.

127 Hope Egan, "Rewire Your Taste Buds—Can You Give God Your Appetite?," *Faith and Fitness Magazine*, December 2009, http://faithandfitness.net/node/2818.

128 Malkmus, *The Hallelujah Diet*, 51.

129 Ibid., 198.

130 Ibid., 51–54.

131 Karl Marx, *Capital*, vol. 1 (London: Penguin Classics, 1990), 165.

132 Malkmus, *The Hallelujah Diet*, 35.

133 Crystal Bowman and Tricia Goyer, *Whit's End Mealtime Devotions: 90 Faith-Building Ideas Your Kids Will Eat Up!* (Carol Stream, IL: Tyndale House, 2013), 24.

134 Ibid.

135 Ibid.

136 Shamblin, *The Weigh Down Diet*, 42.

137 Tanner, *Diets Don't Work*, 88.

138 Hancock, *The Eden Diet*, 94.

139 Tanner, *Diets Don't Work*, 33.

140 Sam Goode, *Why You Should Not Have Sex before Marriage: The Christian Perspective* (Norwalk, CA: Hermit Kingdom Press, 2006), 4.

141 Gregory Jantz, *The Spiritual Path to Weight Loss: Praising God by Living a Healthy Life* (Lincolnwood, IL: Publications International, 2000), 218–220.

142 Chapian and Coyle, *Free to Be Thin*, 21.

143 Weaver, *Fit for God*, 183.

144 Warren et al., *The Daniel Plan*, 77.

145 Adolfo Sagastume, *The Jesus Diet* (n.p. eBook: Amazon Digital Services, 2011).

146 Barbra Sonnen-Hernandez, *The JESUS Diet: Taking the Weight off Your Soul* (Grand Rapids, MI: Zondervan, 2011), 2.

147 Ibid., 5.

3   PRIMITIVE DIETS AND THE "PARADISE PARADOX"

1 Paul Zimmet, "Epidemiology of Diabetes and Its Macrovascular Manifestations in Pacific Populations: The Medical Effects of Social Progress," *Diabetes Care* 2, no. 2 (March 1979): 144–145.

2 S. T. McGarvey, "Obesity in Samoans and a Perspective on Its Etiology in Polynesians," *American Journal of Critical Nutrition* 53, no. 6 (June 1991).

3 Zachary Bloomgarden, "International Diabetes Federation Meeting, 1997," *Diabetes Care* 21, no. 5 (May 1998): 860.

4 Nick Squires, "Obesity Epidemic Destroying Paradise: South Pacific Crisis," *National Post*, February 22, 2007.

5 The Ancestral Health Society, "Manifesto," *About AHS*, http://www.ancestralhealth .org/about.

6 Weston Price, *Nutrition and Physical Degeneration: A Comparison of Primitive and Modern Diets and Their Effects* (New York: P. B. Hoeber, 1939), 59.

7 Susan Yager, *The Hundred Year Diet: America's Voracious Appetite for Losing Weight* (Emmaus, PA: Rodale Press, 2010), 62–65.

8 Vilhjalmur Stefansson, *My Life with the Eskimo* (New York: The Macmillan Company, 1913), 178, 339.

9 Sylvester Graham, *Lectures on the Science of Human Life* (Boston: Marsh, Capen, Lyon, and Webb, 1839), 25.

10 Price, *Nutrition and Physical Degeneration*, 73.

11 Philip Deloria, *Playing Indian* (New Haven, CT: Yale University Press, 1998), 18–19.

12 P. H. Bennett, T. A. Burch, and M. Miller, "Diabetes Mellitus in American (Pima) Indians," *The Lancet* 298, no. 7716 (July 17, 1971): 125.

13 Leslie J. Baier and Robert L. Hanson, "Genetic Studies of the Etiology of Type 2 Diabetes in Pima Indians: Hunting for Pieces to a Complicated Puzzle," *Diabetes* 53, no. 5 (2004): 1181–1186.

14 In unhappy alliance, these two groups are also studied to show how social and political changes increase disease rates among genetically similar populations: the Mexico-U.S.

border that separated Pima Indians and the rural-urban divide in Western Samoa have similarly shaped diabetes trends. Urban Western Samoans have double the diabetes rates of their rural counterparts; American Pimas have rates of 38 percent while their Mexican counterparts had comparatively low incidence rates of 7 percent. Leandris C. Liburd, *Diabetes and Health Disparities: Community-Based Approaches for Racial and Ethnic Populations* (New York: Springer, 2010).

15 Baier and Hanson, "Genetic Studies of the Etiology of Type 2 Diabetes in Pima Indians," 1181.

16 Paul Zimmet, "Globalization, Coca-Colonization and the Chronic Disease Epidemic: Can the Doomsday Scenario Be Averted?," *Journal of Internal Medicine* 247, no. 3 (2000): 309.

17 Renato Rosaldo, "Imperialist Nostalgia," *Representations* 26 (Spring 1989): 107–108.

18 W.J.T. Mitchell, *Landscape and Power* (Chicago: University of Chicago Press, 1994), 10.

19 Price, *Nutrition and Physical Degeneration*, 128.

20 Harvey Levenstein, *Fear of Food: A History of Why We Worry about What We Eat* (Chicago: University of Chicago Press, 2012), 108.

21 Robert McCarrison, *Studies in Deficiency Disease* (London: Henry Frowde and Hodder & Stoughton, 1921), 9. See also McCarrison, "The Nation's Larder in Wartime: Medical Aspects of the Use of Food," *The British Medical Journal* 1, no. 4145 (1940): 984.

22 Shafqat Hussain, *Remoteness and Modernity: Transformation and Continuity in Northern Pakistan* (New Haven, CT: Yale University Press, 2015), 12.

23 Sylvester Graham, *A Lecture to Young Men on Chastity* (Boston: Light & Stearns, Crocker & Brewster, 1837), 155–157.

24 Kyla Wazana Tompkins, *Racial Indigestion: Eating Bodies in the 19th Century* (New York: New York University Press, 2012), 66–67.

25 James Salisbury, *The Relation of Alimentation and Diseases* (New York: J. H. Vail and Co., 1888), 14–15.

26 John Harvey Kellogg, *The Natural Diet of Man* (Battle Creek, MI: Modern Medicine Publishing Company, 1923), 228, 14–15.

27 Jill Nienhiser, "About the Foundation," *The Weston A. Price Foundation*, January 1, 2000, http://www.westonaprice.org/about-us/about-the-foundation/.

28 Ibid.

29 Ancestral Health Society, "Manifesto."

30 Shintani trademarked "HawaiiDiet" in 1997, later renewed in 2001. I refer to *The HawaiiDiet* without a space to indicate the 1997 book published by Pocket Books. The "Hawaii Diet" refers to Shintani's diet plan, promoted both in *The HawaiiDiet* and other media. For trademark application records, please see http://tmsearch.uspto.gov/bin /showfield?f=doc&state=4809:h46duu.2.1.

31 Weight loss averaged 17.1 pounds in the trial but later follow-up studies suggest substantial regain. Few clinical studies have been conducted, with varied success. *Primal Pacific*, a similar New Zealand program, found "wildly unspectacular" results, with "minimal changes and no difference in health outcomes." Terry Shintani, *The HawaiiDiet* (New York: Pocket Books, 1997), xv; Terry Shintani, Sheila Beckham, Helen Kanawaliwali

O'Conner, Claire Hughes, and Alvin Sato, "The Wai'anae Diet Program: A Culturally Sensitive, Community-Based Obesity and Clinical Intervention Program for the Native Hawaiian Population," *Hawaiian Medical Journal* 53, no. 5 (May 1994): 136–137; Mikki Williden, "Primal Pacific: The Efficacy of a Culturally Appropriate LCHF Diet Trial for Reducing Health Risk among Pacific Employees," paper presented at the Ancestral Health Symposium, Berkeley, CA, August 2014.

32 Terry Shintani, letter to author, July 25, 2014. Please see Patrick Vinton Kirch, *Kua'āina Kahiko: Life and Land in Ancient Kahikinui, Maui* (Honolulu: University of Hawaii Press, 2014) for an excellent description of agricultural labor and a refutation of claims for precontact isolation.

33 Terry Shintani, interview with author, June 16, 2014.

34 Shintani, *The HawaiiDiet*, 27.

35 Jessica Hardin and Christina Kwauk, "Producing Markets, Producing People: Local Food, Financial Prosperity and Health in Samoa," *Food, Culture, and Society* 18, no. 3 (2015): 526.

36 Claire Ku'uleilani Hughes, "E ala! E alu! E kuilima!—Up! Together! Join hands!," *Ka Wai Ola* 29, no. 3 (March/Malaki 2012): 20.

37 Neil Sands, "Pacific Nations Battle Obesity Epidemic," *The Independent*, April 11, 2011, http://www.independent.co.uk/life-style/health-and-families/pacific-nations-battle-obesity-epidemic-2266242.html.

38 Dan Hazelwood, "Rising Tide of Diabetes among Pacific Islanders" (Centers for Disease Control and Prevention Podcast), May 2008, http://www2c.cdc.gov/podcasts/media/pdf/RisingTidePI.pdf.

39 Steven Pratt, "Far-Flung Flavors: Looking for the Future of Hawaii's Food in Its Past," *Chicago Tribune*, August 26, 2003; Judith Fitzpatrick-Nietschmann, "Pacific Islanders—Migration and Health," *Western Journal of Medicine* 139, no. 6 (December 1983): 848–853.

40 Hawaii Department of Health, Healthy Hawai'i Initiative, "Obesity in Hawaii Rising alongside National Trends" (press release), August 21, 2013, http://health.hawaii.gov/news/files/2013/05/13-047-Press-Release-F-as-in-Fat.pdf.

41 The Office of Hawaiian Affairs defines "native Hawaiians" by 50 percent native blood quantum, while those with lower quantums are either "Hawaiian" or use the uppercase "N" for "Native Hawaiian." Capitalization conventions are inconsistent: the press release, for example, uses "Native" and "native" interchangeably. Rather than rely on U.S. policy, I follow conventions established by Haunani-Kay Trask to capitalize "Native" to distinguish between immigrants and indigenous peoples. See Haunani-Kay Trask, *From a Native Daughter: Colonialism and Sovereignty in Hawaii* (Monro, ME: Common Courage Press, 1993). See also J. Kēhaulani Kauanui for an assessment of the colonial politics of blood quantum. Kauanui, *Hawaiian Blood: Colonialism and the Politics of Sovereignty and Indigeneity* (Durham, NC: Duke University Press, 2008).

42 Douglas Webb, "Trading Health for Wealth? Obesity in the South Pacific," *United Nations Development Programme*, April 19, 2013, http://www.undp.org/content/undp/en/home/ourperspective/ourperspective-articles/2013/04/19/trading-health-for-wealth-obesity-in-the-south-pacific-doug-webb.html.

43 Medical research regularly cites dwindling numbers of pure Native Hawaiians, perhaps relying on what J. Kēhaulani Kauanui calls the "genocidal logic" and "romantic desire for extinction" that ignores the rising numbers of all Hawaiian people by "obsessing over the so-called full-bloods." In New Zealand, a government website has announced an expert's "warn[ing] that diabetes could wipe out Māori and Pacific Islanders by the end of the century." A 2007 *Journal of the CardioMetabolic Syndrome* article is representative of medical reports. The second paragraph chronicles eighteenth- and nineteenth-century population decline, summarizing projections that "no full-blood Native Hawaiians will remain in 2045." Later in the study, the authors assert: "Increases in obesity, heart disease, and diabetes among Native Hawaiians also have been attributed to changes in key lifestyle practices resulting from rapid 'westernization'—including reduced physical activity and changes from a traditional diet." Since the "islands of Hawaii are the most isolated lands in the world," the authors suggest, the "broad legacy of losses following Western contact" are particularly acute. In response, activists note that the traditional "low-fat, high-fiber diet has helped combat two modern ailments—obesity and diabetes—that are killing many Native Hawaiians." Kauanui, *Hawaiian Blood*, 16; Noa Emmett Aluli, Phillip W. Reyes, and JoAnn 'Umilani Tsark, "Cardiovascular Disease Disparities in Native Hawaiians," *Journal of the CardioMetabolic Syndrome* 2, no. 4 (Fall 2007): 252; Meki Cox, "Hawaiians Find Better Health in Roots," *Los Angeles Times*, July 28, 1996, http://articles.latimes.com/1996-07-28/news/mn-28787 _1_native-hawaiians.

44 Tom Dye, "Population Trends in Hawaii before 1778," *Hawaiian Journal of History* 28 (1994): 1–20.

45 "Profile: Native Hawaiians and Pacific Islanders," *Office of Minority Health*, February 17, 2017, https://minorityhealth.hhs.gov/omh/browse.aspx?lvl=3&lvlid=65.

46 Barrie Macdonald, "'Now an Island Is Too Big': Limits and Limitations of Pacific Islands History," *Journal of Pacific Studies* 20 (1996): 20–27.

47 Paul Jaminet and Shou-Ching Jaminet, *Perfect Health Diet: Regain Health and Lose Weight by Eating the Way You Were Meant to Eat* (New York: Scribner, 2012), 238.

48 Spencer Wells, *Pandora's Seed: Why the Hunter-Gatherer Holds the Key to Our Survival* (New York: Random House, 2011), 68.

49 Sunia Foliaki and Neil Pearce, "Prevalence and Causes of Diabetes in Pacific Populations," *Pacific Health Dialog* 10, no. 2 (2003): 90.

50 Neal Barnard, *The 21-Day Weight Loss Kickstart* (New York: Grand Central Life & Style, 2011).

51 Cherie Calbom and John Calbom, *The Coconut Diet* (New York: Warner Books, 2005); Lisa Dorfman, *The Tropical Diet: A Scientific, Simple, & Sexy Weight Loss Strategy* (Miami, FL: Food Fitness International, 2004), xiv. Emphasis in original.

52 For the artistic response to these diseases, see the poetry of Craig Santos Perez and Dan Taulapapa McMullin. Deborah Madsen, *The Routledge Companion to Native American Literature* (New York: Routledge, 2015), 50.

53 Jaminet and Jaminet, *Perfect Health Diet*, xi.

54 Brij V. Lal and Kate Fortune, "Fatal Impact," in *The Pacific Islands: An Encyclopedia* (Honolulu: University of Hawaii Press, 2000), 83–85.

55 Oliver Bennett, *Cultural Pessimism: Narratives of Decline in the Postmodern World* (Edinburgh: Edinburgh University Press, 2001).

56 Scholarship on the Pacific Islands is critical to understanding the currency of the precontact diet. Cari Costanzo Kapur's study of memory and the quest for Native Hawaiian rights, together with Jocelyn Linnekin and Richard Handler's analysis of invented tradition, helps illuminate the active memory- and identity-making processes of the narratives. Jean Kim's history of dental experiments and "imperial nutrition" in the first half of the twentieth century helps historicize diet-based disease in Hawaii. Structural anthropological and neo-Darwinist ideas of fatal impact theory elucidate the relationship between diabetes and colonization. Rob Wilson's call for a complex, changing, and hybrid inside-out Pacific-centered methodology pertains to diet advice which often depends on the outside-in assessment of the diseased, docile Native body. Also relevant is Albert Wendt's refutation of the *"noble savage* literary school" and the totalizing stereotypes of the Pacific Islands in Western literature, which imagine the Islands as Edenic paradises and portray Islanders as "stereotyped childlike pagan[s] who need to be steered to the Light." Cari Costanzo Kapur, "Rights, Roots, and Resistance: Land and Indigenous (trans)Nationalism in Contemporary Hawai'i," PhD diss., Stanford University, 2005; Handler and Linnekin, "Tradition, Genuine or Spurious"; Jean Kim, "Experimental Encounters: Filipino and Hawaiian Bodies in the U.S. Imperial Invention of Odontoclasia," *American Quarterly* 63, no. 2 (September 2010): 523–546; Rob Wilson, "Introduction: Toward Imagining a New Pacific," in *Inside Out: Literature, Cultural Politics, and Identity in the New Pacific,* ed. Vilsoni Hereniko and Rob Wilson (Oxford: Rowman and Littlefield, 1999), 4; Albert Wendt, "Towards a New Oceania," *Mana Review* 1, no. 1 (1976): 49–60. Emphasis in original.

57 Gary Paul Nabhan, *Why Some Like It Hot: Food, Genes, and Cultural Diversity* (Washington, DC: Island Press/Shearwater Books, 2004), 207–209. Emphasis in original.

58 Ibid., 209. Emphasis in original.

59 Senator John Henry Wise, a Native politician, used the diet-health relationship to support the Hawaiian Homelands Act of 1921. In a 1920 interview, Wise explained that the "Hawaiian people are a dying people … Some attribute it to liquor, some to disease, and some to the mode of living. Now the taro, the Hawaiian food, was the only food they had for generations outside of sweet potatoes. When civilization came into the country other foods were brought in." By repatriating the "lands back to the Hawaiians," Wise believed traditional foods and mode of living could help rehabilitate the race. Theodore M. Knappen, "The Hawaiian Race Threatened with Extinction," *New York Tribune,* June 13, 1920: F2; "Hawaiian Race Vanishing, Says U.S. Naturalist," *San Francisco Chronicle,* April, 11, 1920: W4.

60 Price, *Nutrition and Physical Degeneration,* 85–87.

61 Rosaldo, "Imperialist Nostalgia," 108.

62 Paul Bragg, *Healthful Eating without Confusion* (Desert Hot Springs, CA: Health Science, 1976), 9–11.

63 Theodore Dalrymple, "A Lesson from the Pacific," *New Statesman* 15, no. 724 (September 16, 2002); Paul Zimmet, Gary Dowse, Caroline Finch, Sue Serjeantson, and Hilary King, "The Epidemiology and Natural History of NIDDM—Lessons from the South Pacific," *Diabetes/Metabolism Research and Reviews* 6 (1990): 91–124.

64 Zimmet, "Globalization, Coca-Colonization and the Chronic Disease Epidemic," 302.

65 Doug Munro and Brij V. Lal, *Texts and Contexts: Reflections in Pacific Islands Historiography* (Honolulu: University of Hawaii Press, 2006), 35.

66 David Stannard, "The Hawaiians: Health, Justice, and Sovereignty," *Cultural Survival Quarterly* 24, no. 1 (2000).

67 Robert George Hughes, *Diet, Food Supply, and Obesity in the Pacific* (Manila, Philippines: World Health Organization, Regional Office for the Western Pacific, 2003), 16.

68 Ibid., 40.

69 Shintani et al., "The Wai'anae Diet Program," 136.

70 As Rachel Laudan notes in her 1996 culinary history of Hawaii, blended recipes like these better represent the diversity of "local" cuisine. Rachel Laudan, *The Food of Paradise: Exploring Hawaii's Culinary Heritage* (Honolulu: The University of Hawaii Press, 1996), 31.

71 Shintani, interview, June 16, 2014.

72 Shintani, *The HawaiiDiet*, 4.

73 Dorfman, *The Tropical Diet*, 3.

74 Nabhan, *Why Some Like It Hot*, 210.

75 Shintani, *The HawaiiDiet*, 6.

76 Wilson, "Introduction: Toward Imagining a New Pacific," 2.

77 Shintani et al., "The Wai'anae Diet Program," 35.

78 Echoing W.J.T. Mitchell's claim that landscape could be seen as the "'dreamwork' of imperialism," Jill Casid traces how the colonial project harnessed an Emersonian understanding of the transcendental power of a pure landscape. European empire, Casid argues, "reformulated itself as its opposite, an anti-empire, by putting botany in the central place." Celebrating nature of course instrumentalizes and misuses Emerson's legacy, and revering the landscape may not simply be a harmless dream of an alternative past but a necessary vision attendant to the naturalization of empire. Much of Pacific Islands diet advice venerates precontact landscapes as cures for postcolonial disease, revealing the tenacity of the long transcendentalist tradition entwining body, land, and spirit. For example, Shintani claims in a section called "Tragic Irony" that "the inherent healthiness of the land remains" and by eating "in harmony with nature" and the "spirit of aloha," dieters will lose weight. W.J.T. Mitchell, *Landscape and Power*, 10; Jill H. Casid, *Sowing Empire: Landscape and Colonization* (Minneapolis: University of Minnesota Press, 2005), 240; Shintani, *The HawaiiDiet*, 15.

79 Takaaki Nishiyama, "Nauru: An Island Plagued by Obesity and Diabetes," *The Asahi Shimbun Globe*, May 27, 2012, http://ajw.asahi.com/article/globe/feature/obesity/AJ2 01205270051.

80 Kathy Marks, "Fat of the Land: Nauru Tops Obesity League," *The Independent*, December 26, 2010, http://www.independent.co.uk/life-style/health-and-families /health-news/fat-of-the-land-nauru-tops-obesity-league-2169418.html.

81 Juliet McMullin, "The Call to Life: Revitalizing a Healthy Hawaiian Identity," *Social Science and Medicine* 61 (2005): 809–820, 820.

82 To protest deplorable conditions, refugees have also self-immolated in front of UN cameras. Roger Cohen, "Broken Men in Paradise," *The New York Times*, December 9, 2016.

83 Terry Shintani and Claire Ku'uleilani Hughes, *The Wai'anae Book of Hawaiian Health* (Wai'anae, HI: Wai'anae Coast Comprehensive Health Center, 1991), 2.

84 Shintani, interview, June 16, 2014.

85 Lyman Tower Sargent, "The Three Faces of Utopianism Revisited," *Utopian Studies* 5, no. 1 (1994): 1–37; Sargent, *Utopianism: A Very Short Introduction* (New York: Oxford University Press, 2010), 4.

86 Shintani, *The HawaiiDiet*, 263–264.

87 Richard Handler and Jocelyn Linnekin, "Tradition, Genuine or Spurious," *The Journal of American Folklore* 97, no. 385 (September 1984): 273–290.

88 Eric Hobsbawm and Terence Ranger, eds., *The Invention of Tradition* (Cambridge: Cambridge University Press, 1983).

89 Seven years after he published *The History of Sexuality* in 1976, Michel Foucault argued that prohibitions against food were also instrumental in creating a sense of the modern self: a self perceived as a self-regulating, autonomous subject that could control the needs of the body and the direction of the mind. Michel Foucault, "On the Genealogy of Ethics: An Overview of a Work in Progress," in *Michel Foucault: Beyond Structuralism and Hermeneutics*, ed. Hubert Dreyfus and Paul Rabinow (Chicago: University of Chicago Press, 1983), 229.

90 Handler and Linnekin, "Tradition, Genuine or Spurious," 276.

91 Shintani, interview, June 16, 2014.

92 Kauila Clark, qtd. in Daphne Miller and Allison Sarubin-Fragakis, *The Jungle Effect: A Doctor Discovers the Healthiest Diets from around the World* (New York: Collins, 2008), 53.

93 See J. Kēhaulani Kauanui, *Hawaiian Blood*, for an insightful intervention in the narratives of civilization, upending the "authenticity" of blood quantum requirements and deftly demonstrating how blood-based racialization served the colonial project to diminish claims for sovereignty and political power.

94 Kapur, "Rights, Roots, and Resistance," 190.

95 Ibid., 189.

96 Ranajit Guha and Gayatri Chakravorty Spivak, *Selected Subaltern Studies* (New York: Oxford University Press, 1988).

97 Shintani interview, June 16, 2014.

98 Geoffrey White and Ty P. Kāwika Tengan, "Disappearing Worlds: Anthropology and Cultural Studies in Hawai'i and the Pacific," *Contemporary Pacific* 13, no. 2 (Fall 2001): 388.

99 James Clifford, *Routes: Travel and Translation in the Late Twentieth Century* (Cambridge, MA: Harvard University Press, 1997), 4.

100 Hokulani K. Aikau, "Indigeneity in the Diaspora: The Case of Native Hawaiians at Iosepa, Utah," *American Quarterly* 62, no. 3 (2010): 478.

101 Carolyn Mein, *Different Bodies, Different Diets: Discover a Health and Diet Plan That Fits You* (New York: Regan Books, 2001); Marie Savard, with Carol Svec, *The Body Shape Solution to Weight Loss and Wellness: The Apples & Pears Approach to Losing Weight, Living Longer, and Feeling Healthier* (New York: Atria Books, 2005).

102 Patricia Vertinsky, "Embodying Normalcy: Anthropometry and the Long Arm of William H. Sheldon's Somatotyping Project," *Journal of Sport History* 29, no. 1 (2002): 97.

103 Peter D'Adamo and Catherine Whitney, *Eat Right 4 Your Type: The Individualized Diet Solution to Staying Healthy, Living Longer, and Achieving Your Ideal Weight* (New York: G. P. Putnam's Sons, 1996), xiv–xv.

104 Ibid., 12.

105 Louise Williams and Peter Williams, "Evaluation of a Tool for Rating Popular Diet Books," *Nutrition and Dietetics* 60, no. 3 (2003): 185–197.

106 Peter D'Adamo, with Catherine Whitney, *Eat Right 4 Your Type: The Individualized Blood Type Diet Solution* (New York: Berkley Press, 2016), xii.

107 Sharon Moalem, *The DNA Restart: Unlock Your Personal Genetic Code to Eat for Your Genes, Lose Weight, and Reverse Aging* (Emmaus, PA: Rodale Press, 2016), xiv–xv.

108 Ibid., 1.

109 Reginald Horsman, *The New Republic: The United States of America 1789-1815* (New York: Routledge, 2000), 138.

110 Samuel Stanhope Smith, *An Essay on the Causes of the Variety of Complexion and Figure in the Human Species* (New Brunswick, NJ: J. Simpson and Co, 1810), 150, in the Hathi Trust Digital Library, https://babel.hathitrust.org/cgi/pt?id=pst.000006225438.

111 Ibid., 165.

112 Bob Kuska, "Breast Cancer Increases on Papua New Guinea," *Journal of the National Cancer Institute* 91, no. 12 (1999): 994–996.

113 James Clifford and George E. Marcus, *Writing Culture: The Poetics and Politics of Ethnography* (Berkeley: University of California Press, 1986), 101.

114 Ibid., 113.

115 Renato Rosaldo, "From the Door of His Tent: The Fieldworker and the Inquisitor," in *Writing Culture: The Poetics and Politics of Ethnography*, ed. James Clifford and George Marcus (Berkeley: University of California Press, 1986), 91.

116 Paul Zimmet, "Epidemiology of Diabetes and Its Macrovascular Manifestations in Pacific Populations," 144–145.

117 Joshua Keating, "Why Do the World's Fattest People Live on Islands?," *Foreign Policy*, February 9, 2011, http://foreignpolicy.com/2011/02/09/why-do-the-worlds-fattest-people-live-on-islands/.

118 Sander Gilman. *Obesity: The Biography* (Oxford: Oxford University Press, 2010), 159.

119 Qtd. in Sander Gilman, *Diets and Dieting: A Cultural Encyclopedia* (New York: Routledge, 2008), 195.

120 Zimmet, "Epidemiology of Diabetes and Its Macrovascular Manifestations in Pacific Populations," 148.

121 Michael Curtis, "The Obesity Epidemic in the Pacific," *Journal of Development and Social Transformation* 1 (November 2004): 38.

122 R. R. Thaman, "Consumerism, the Media, and Malnutrition in the Pacific Islands," *Pacific Health Dialog* 10, no. 1 (2003): 86.

123 "Lifestyle Disease Situation out of Control," *Islands Business*, February 2014, http://www.islandsbusiness.com/2014/2/we-say/lifestyle-disease-situation-out-of-control/.

124 Paul Lyons, *American Pacificism: Oceania in the U.S. Imagination* (New York: Routledge, 2006), 137–140.

125 Qtd. in ibid., 135.

126 Charles Hanley, "Pacific Islanders Top the Scales," *The Charleston Gazette*, May 10, 2004.

127 Curtis, "The Obesity Epidemic in the Pacific," 39.

128 George Lewis, "From Minnesota Fat to Seoul Food: Spam in America and the Pacific Rim," *The Journal of Popular Culture* 34, no. 2 (Fall 2000): 83–105.

129 Deborah B. Gewertz and Frederick Karl Errington, *Cheap Meat: Flap Food Nations in the Pacific Islands* (Berkeley: University of California Press, 2010), 4.

130 Merrill Singer, "Following the Turkey Tails: Neoliberal Globalization and the Political Ecology of Health," *Journal of Political Ecology* 21 (2014): 436–451.

131 Mike Seccombe, "Bum Deal on Back End of Big Birds," *The Global Mail*, November 19, 2013, http://www.theglobalmail.org/feature/bum-deal-on-back-end-of-big-birds/483/.

132 Paul Theroux, qtd. in Paul Lyons, "From Man-Eaters to Spam-Eaters: Literary Tourism and the Discourse of Cannibalism from Herman Melville to Paul Theroux," *Multiculturalism and Representation: Selected Essays*, ed. John Rieder and Larry E. Smith (Honolulu: University of Hawaii Press, 1996), 77.

133 Augustus Earle, qtd. in Geoffrey Sanborn, *The Sign of the Cannibal: Melville and the Making of a Postcolonial Reader* (Durham, NC: Duke University Press, 1998), 5.

134 J. C. Furnas, *Anatomy of Paradise: Hawaii and the Islands of the South Seas* (New York: William Sloane Associates, 1948), 79. Emphasis in original.

135 Douglas Oliver, *The Pacific Islands* (Cambridge, MA: Harvard University Press, 1951), 21.

136 Robert Siegel, "Samoans Await the Return of the Tasty Turkey Tail," *NPR: All Things Considered*, May 9, 2013, http://www.npr.org/blogs/thesalt/2013/05/14/182568333/samoans-await-the-return-of-the-tasty-turkey-tail.

137 Susan Cassels, "Overweight in the Pacific: Links between Foreign Dependence, Global Food Trade, and Obesity in the Federated States of Micronesia," *Globalization and Health* 2, no. 10 (2006).

138 Squires, "Obesity Epidemic Destroying Paradise."

139 Stefan Gates, "Trouble in Paradise," *The Guardian*, August 2, 2006.

140 Squires, "Obesity Epidemic Destroying Paradise."

141 Gates, "Trouble in Paradise."

142 Robyn McDermott, "Ethics, Epidemiology and the Thrifty Gene: Biological Determinism as a Health Hazard," *Social Science & Medicine* 47, no. 9 (November 1998): 1189–1195.

143 Herman Melville, *Typee: A Peep at Polynesian Life*, ed. Harrison Hayford, Hershel Parker, and G. Thomas Tanselle (Chicago: Northwestern University Press, 1968), 124.

144 Gates, "Trouble in Paradise."

145 Webb, "Trading Health for Wealth?"

4 DETOXIFICATION DIETS AND CONCEPTS OF A TOXIC MODERNITY

1 Saguy, *What's Wrong with Fat?* (New York: Oxford University Press, 2013), 6.

2 Chin Jou, "The Biology and Genetics of Obesity—A Century of Inquiries," *New England Journal of Medicine* 2014, no. 370 (May 15, 2014): 1874–1877.

3 Merla Zellerbach, with Phyllis Saifer, *Detox: A Successful & Supportive Program for Freeing Your Body from the Physical and Psychological Effects of Chemical Pollutants (at Home & at Work), Junk Food Additives, Sugar, Nicotine, Drugs, Alcohol, Caffeine, Prescription and Nonprescription Medications, and Other Environmental Toxins* (Los Angeles: J. P. Tarcher, 1984), 56.

4 Ibid., 24.

5 M. Discipulo, interview by author, Stanford, CA, March 12, 2015.

6 Peter Pressman, qtd. in Abby Ellin, "Flush Those Toxins! Eh, Not So Fast," *The New York Times*, January 7, 2014, http://www.nytimes.com/2009/01/22/fashion/22skin.html?partner=rss.

7 Knowles famously lost twenty pounds doing the "Master Cleanse" fasting diet of lemon juice, maple syrup, and cayenne pepper to prepare for the 2006 *Dreamgirls* film. In 2008, Winfrey promoted her twenty-one-day weight loss detox program after her much-touted weight loss. Hayek branded a detoxification "cooler cleanse" and edible moisturizer line inspired by her grandmother's Mexican beauty secrets.

8 Peter Pressman, "Flush Those Toxins!"

9 Connie Diekman, qtd. in Melody Kemp, "Extinction in a Bottle," *Global Times*, May 20, 2013, http://www.globaltimes.cn/content/782743.shtml.

10 Roni DeLuz, *21 Pounds in 21 Days: The Martha's Vineyard Diet Detox* (New York: Harper Collins, 2007).

11 Mark Hyman, *The Blood Sugar Solution 10-Day Detox Diet: Activate Your Body's Natural Ability to Burn Fat and Lose Weight Fast* (New York: Little, Brown, 2014), 9.

12 Zellerbach, *Detox*, 124.

13 Ibid., 5.

14 Rachel Carson, *Silent Spring* (Boston: Houghton Mifflin, 1962), 20.

15 Zellerbach, *Detox*, 181.

16 Ibid., 2.

17 Ibid., 147–148.

18 William Dufty, *Sugar Blues* (Radnor, PA: Chilton Book Co., 1975), 12.

19 Mary Daniels, "Gloria Urges, Quit Taking Your Lumps of Sugar," *Chicago Tribune*, April 11, 1976.

20 Theron Randolph, "The Descriptive Features of Food Addiction: Addictive Eating and Drinking," *Quarterly Journal of Studies on Alcohol* 17, no. 2 (1956): 198–224.

21 John Opie, *Nature's Nation: An Environmental History of the United States* (Fort Worth, TX: Harcourt, 1998), 416–417.

22 Mark Jackson, *Allergy: The History of a Modern Malady* (London: Reaktion, 2006), 202.

23 Lisa M. Ortigara Crego, "The Experience of a Spiritual Recovery from Food Addiction: A Heuristic Inquiry" (PhD diss., Capella University, 2006), 2.

24 In 2009, Yale Medical School introduced a widely used "food addiction scale" test to determine whether patients suffered from the addiction.

25 Zellerbach, *Detox*, 128–129.

26 Ibid., 129.

27 U.S. Department of Health and Human Services, *Overweight and Obesity Statistics*, http://www.niddk.nih.gov/health-information/health-statistics/Documents/stat904z.pdf.

28 John Fekner, "Toxic Junkie Text Entry," *Research Archive*, 2010, http://johnfekner.com/feknerArchive/?p=1249#more-1249.

29 Pat Inglis, "Gloria Swanson Talks of Food, Not Films," *The Montreal Gazette*, August 23, 1977, 19.

30 David Fertig, *Analogy and Morphological Change* (Edinburgh: Edinburgh University Press, 2013), 24.

31 Laura McCarthy, "Born Losers: The New Diet Junkies," *Mademoiselle: The Magazine for the Smart Young Woman* 94 (1988): 156.

32 Renée Taylor, *My Life on a Diet: Confessions of a Hollywood Diet Junkie* (New York: Putnam, 1986).

33 Art Mollen, *The Mollen Method: A 30-Day Program to Lifetime Health Addiction* (Emmaus, PA: Rodale Press, 1986), 24.

34 Glenn O'Brien, "All about Madonna," *Interview Magazine*, June 1990, http://allaboutmadonna.com/madonna-library/madonna-interview-interview-magazine-june-1990.

35 Elizabeth Sharon Hayenga, "Dieting through the Decades: A Comparative Study of Weight Reduction in America as Depicted in Popular Literature and Books from 1940 to the Late 1980s" (PhD diss., University of Minnesota, 1989), 103.

36 Deborah DeEugenio and Debra Henn, *Diet Pills* (Philadelphia: Chelsea House, 2005), 46–48.

37 "Suit In Fen-Phen Death Ends with Settlement," *Philadelphia Inquirer* (Inquirer Wire Services), January 28, 2000, http://articles.philly.com/2000-01-28/business/25596888_1_fen-phen-diet-drug-combination-pondimin.

38 "Kitty Dukakis Admits Addiction to Diet Pills for 26 Years," *Orlando Sentinel*, July 9, 1987, A4.

39 Nicolas Rasmussen, *On Speed: The Many Lives of Amphetamine* (New York: New York University Press, 2008), 239.

40 "Detox Diet Is Key to a Sizzling Summer," *The Mirror* (London), June 29, 1999, 20.

41 Carmel Allen, "The 72-Hour Hangover Cure: Start a Detox Diet Today for a Clean Break before the New Year Binge," *Mail on Sunday*, December 27, 1998, 45.

42 One British author named Jane Scrivner fed a seemingly insatiable British appetite for detox diet books by publishing six books in the space of two years. Between 1999 and 2001, she published *Detox Your Mind, Detox Your Life, The Little Book of Detox, Jane Scrivner's Total Detox: 6 Ways to Revitalise Your Life, Stay Young: Detox*, and *Detox Your Hangover: 99 Ways to Feel 100% Better*. Each of her books offered a slightly different approach, but all used a short-term detox program to rid the body of alcohol and other addictive substances. Jane Scrivner, "Clean Break," *The Times of India*, January 24, 1998, 1.

43 Elson Haas, *The Detox Diet: A How and When-to Guide for Cleansing the Body* (Berkeley, CA: Celestial Arts, 1996), 57.

44 Asa Hershoff, *Homeopathic Remedies: A Quick and Easy Guide to Common Disorders and Their Homeopathic Treatments* (Garden City Park, NY: Avery Publishing Group, 1999), 82.

45 The "toxic soup" of American life has long informed drug and alcohol treatment in the United States. As far back as the eighteenth century, American addicts were given the quarantine cure—isolating addicts into asylums, live-in centers, retreats, halfway homes, agricultural colonies, and shelters. Many treatment centers were rural or particularly picturesque, promising better health through open vistas, pure air, and distance from the clamor and crime of modern living. The New York State Inebriate Asylum is particularly memorable. Established in 1858, the stone and brick building was celebrated at the time for its Tudor castellated style and its "beautiful elevated site" of 250 acres. Illustrations of the asylum highlight its bucolic elements, showing reformed addicts scything grass or taking their morning constitutionals. Other asylums were also noted for their beauty, like the 1882 Martha Washington Home for inebriate women situated on ten picturesque acres in Lake View, Chicago. Located in a "wonderfully charming spot," reporters gushed over the home's shady groves and pleasant temperatures. Presaging the transition to private detox spas, nineteenth-century entrepreneurs such as Edward Mann established private for-profit asylums for the well-to-do drunkard. In 1878, Mann advertised his Sunnyside asylum with promises of billiards, rowing, and horseback riding, as well as "handsomely furnished apartments." Detox centers today are painted in similar terms. Sarah W. Tracy, *Alcoholism in America: From Reconstruction to Prohibition* (Baltimore: Johns Hopkins University Press, 2005).

46 "Detoxify" and "detoxicate" are both older nineteenth-century words with specific toxicological meaning: "to deprive a substance of its poisonous attributes." The liver, for example, naturally detoxicates the blood. The term was not abbreviated until the 1970s, when "detox" was used colloquially to describe the treatment of alcoholics and drug addicts. "Rehab" was also shortened from "rehabilitation" treatment at this time but, unlike detox, rehab more often meant the longer-term, gradual treatment of addiction through behavioral modification, psychological counseling, and medical treatment. Rehab also might involve outpatient treatment whereas detox quickly came to mean a physical place—a center set away from the cities, a place of solitude and ease.

47 P. J. Corkery, "Addiction à L.A. Mode," *New Republic*, July 7, 1985, http://www.newre public.com/article/politics/91735/betty-ford-center-addiction-elizabeth-taylor.

48 Deborah Blumenthal, "A Day in the Life of the Betty Ford Center," *The New York Times*, February 27, 1987, 1.

49 Diane Reischel, "Betty Ford Center Fete Rates in Glitz, Glamour," *Los Angeles Times*, October 21, 1986, 2.

50 Ray Recchi, "Semantic Shenanigans as Low as You Can Go," *Sun Sentinel*, March 27, 1989, 1D.

51 Legs McNeil, "Yuppie Like Me," *Spin* 4, no. 9 (1988), 118, 94.

52 Julie Guthman, *Weighing In: Obesity, Food Justice, and the Limits of Capitalism* (Berkeley: University of California Press, 2011), 18.

53 Charlotte Biltekoff, *Eating Right in America: The Cultural Politics of Food and Health* (Durham, NC: Duke University Press, 2013), 92.

54 Detox diet spas are even more plush. Common services include massage, colonics, ionic footbaths, and lymphatic drainage treatments. Most serve detox meals of fresh juices, spring water, and vegetables while limiting sugar, dairy, wheat, and meat. Day spas also use the language of retreat and vacation to advertise their detox services. DTOX, a midrange day spa in Los Angeles, called their signature package an "urban retreat" and included an herbal tub soak, a body wrap, and a DTOX custom massage for $260. A spa industry spokesperson explained to *Newsweek* in 2008 that upmarket detoxers are "tired of overeating, drinking, and partying too much." "Luxury detox boot camp travel [is] one of the hottest trends in the hospitality industry," as the wealthy prefer detox spas that require giving up sweets, alcohol, and meat. He summarizes: "They've got their wealth and now they want their health." Marc Margolis, "Paying for a Chance to Suffer in Silence," *Newsweek*, May 26, 2008.

55 Paul Bragg and Patricia Bragg, *The Miracle of Fasting Proven throughout History for Physical, Mental, & Spiritual Rejuvenation* (Santa Barbara, CA: Health Science, 1985), 7.

56 Michael Brown, "Can You Detox Your Body?," *American Health* 5 (1986): 56, 53.

57 Jennifer La Forte, "Internal Cleansing & Detoxification," *Yoga Journal*, January– February 1997, 93.

58 Ibid., 93–108.

59 Katie Robinson, "The Secret Meaning of the Lotus Flower," *Town and Country Magazine*, April 28, 2017, http://www.townandcountrymag.com/leisure/arts-and-culture /a9550430/lotus-flower-meaning/.

60 Alternative music took another shot at yuppie detox plans ten years later. In 1998, an English new wave pop band named Heaven 17 released an album cheekily titled *Retox/ Detox*. A review explained that the album summarized "the era's art-school-politico pretensions" with songs like "Crushed by the Wheels (of Industry)" and "(We Don't Need This) Fascist Groove Thang."

61 When specified, the concept of toxins has been defined capaciously and creatively. Over the last hundred years, detoxers have categorized the following as toxic: frying pans, drinking water, apples, potatoes, noise, dust, bright lights, all chemicals, all drugs, flour, sugar, wheat, restaurant food, polyester, nylon, dental fillings, tooth brushes, and wood. Emotional toxins include stress, apathy, jealousy, greed, anxiety, and perfectionism. A *Social Detox* zine circulated in 2007 as "a resource for anti-sexist men" to combat gender privilege and "detox the pyramids of patriarchal power." There are also dozens of "detox" plans for toxic finances, relationships, and homes. Over the last ten years, the detoxification metaphor has been applied to love addicts, porn addicts, and those suffering from cluttered desks and tangled finances. Titles include *Detox Your Finances* (2004), *Detox Your Spiritual Life* (2007), *Sexual Detox: A Guide for Guys Who Are Sick of Porn* (2010), *Detox Your Desk: Declutter Your Life and Mind* (2010), *The 30-Day Dating Detox* (2011), *The Girly Thoughts 10-Day Detox Plan* (2014), and *Insecurity Detox* (2016).

62 Norine Dworkin, "Seasonal Detox: Supercharge Your Health with a Personal Purification Program," *Vegetarian Times*, March 1999, 46.

63 Josie Vertz, interview by author, September 12, 2016, San Francisco, CA.

64 Discipulo, interview.

65 Richard Saltus, "Some Scientists Skeptical of an Obesity Cure," *Boston Globe*, July 28, 1995, 3.

66 Jou, "The Biology and Genetics of Obesity," 1874.

67 Jane Brody, "Personal Health," *The New York Times*, December 25, 1996, C6.

68 F. Xavier Pi-Sunyer, qtd. in Milt Freudenheim, "Employers Focus on Weight as Workplace Health Issue: Medical Costs Rising as Nation Gets Heavier," *The New York Times*, September 6, 1999, A15.

69 Tom Teepen, "Commentary: Americans Live in 'Toxic Food Environment,'" *Dayton Daily News*, March 12, 2004, A10.

70 Hyman, *The Blood Sugar Solution 10-Day Detox Diet*, 69.

71 Jamieson addressed the clinical and addiction roots of the word "detox," explaining that the "concept of detoxing is pretty intense." She elaborates that "most of us equate it with kicking drugs or alcohol, and the word invokes images of people writhing on beds riding out delirium tremens . . . or locked up in prisonlike detox centers." Jamieson agrees that detoxing is still intense but comforts readers that detoxing is also a "gentle method of cleansing and noninvasive way of rebalancing." "Gentle" and "noninvasive" don't exactly describe the previous image of writhing with withdrawal symptoms in prisonlike centers. Effectively, Jamieson denies detox's debts to drug and alcohol addiction treatment and minimizes the torment of drug addiction detox. She avers that "we have become so sugar-dependent that giving it up is just as hard as giving up any drug." Alex Jamieson, *The Great American Detox Diet: 8 Weeks to Weight Loss and Well-Being* (Emmaus, PA: Rodale Press, 2005), 33–34, 69.

72 Ibid., 26–28.

73 Ibid., 24.

74 Jamieson and Spurlock were inspired by a high-profile 2002 lawsuit filed by two obese teenagers against McDonald's, suing the franchise for failing to provide enough information about the nutritional risks of their foods. The case made headlines and raised essential questions about whether a restaurant could be held responsible for

obesity and whether children deserved legal protection from a toxic food environment. The teenagers' lawyer, Samuel Hirsch, stated: "Young individuals are not in a position to make a choice after the onslaught of advertising and promotions," referencing that a typical meal of a Big Mac, super-sized fries, and a super-sized Coke weighs in at 1,600 calories, or more than half of the recommended 2,000–2,200 daily caloric intake for teenage girls. Marc Santora, "Teenagers' Suit Says McDonald's Made Them Obese," *The New York Times*, November 21, 2002; Jamieson, *The Great American Detox Diet*, 25–27.

75 Jamieson, *The Great American Detox Diet*, 27.

76 Ibid., 127.

77 Michael Pollan, *The Omnivore's Dilemma: A Natural History of Four Meals* (New York: Penguin, 2006), 12.

78 Jamieson, *The Great American Detox Diet*, 24.

79 After seeing calorie counts posted prominently on menus, some diners actually increased consumption, assuming that more is better or that low-calorie means less tasty. Others show that some diners, particularly women, decrease calories but, on the whole, the results of menu labeling were deemed insignificant. United States Department of Agriculture Nutrition Evidence Library, *Scientific Report of the 2015 Dietary Guidelines Advisory Committee*, https://health.gov/dietaryguidelines/2015-scientific-report/08-chapter-3/d3-7.asp, 8.

80 Restaurant industry leaders recommend "stealth marketing" instead, following the well-publicized 2007 example of the Starbucks switch from their whole milk to 2 percent dairy standard. By making a lower-calorie option a default, restaurants will actually decrease consumption without relying on active consumer choice. Federal requirements for mandatory labeling are now in limbo as the Affordable Care Act sinks in the Trump administration and these mixed-result studies may also impede their enforcement. Kathleen Meister and Marjorie Doyle, *Obesity and Food Technology* (New York: American Council on Science and Health, 2009), 25.

81 Megan Kimble, "I Gave Up Processed Foods for a Year and This Is What Happened," *Shape*, June 22, 2015, http://www.shape.com/healthy-eating/diet-tips/i-gave-processed -foods-year-and-what-happened.

82 Josée Johnston and Shyon Baumann, *Foodies: Democracy and Distinction in the Gourmet Foodscape* (New York: Routledge, 2009), 119–120.

83 Daniel Fromson, "The New Yorker Weighs In on the Foodie Elitism Debate," *The Atlantic*, July 15, 2010, www.theatlantic.com/health/archive/2010/07/the-new-yorker -weighs-in-on-the-foodie-elitism-debate/59815/.

84 Rhonda Byrne, *The Secret* (New York: Atria Books, 2006).

85 Beryl Satter, *Each Mind a Kingdom: American Women, Sexual Purity, and the New Thought Movement, 1875–1920* (Berkeley: University of California Press, 1999), 3.

86 Jamieson, *The Great American Detox Diet*, 162.

87 Wishful thinking is also a trope picked up specifically by diet books, most notably in the popular 1996 *Think Yourself Thin* that promised to show "dieters how to use the power of their subconscious mind . . . transforming their fantasies of having the perfect

body into reality." Other books followed the law of attraction theme, like the 2009 *You Can Think Yourself Thin*, 2012 *Think and Grow Thin*, and 2015 *Visualization for Weight Loss*. Just around the same time, Barbara Ehrenreich argued more broadly that positive thinking unjustly blames the individual for larger social ills. Rather than looking at larger social or economic forces, positive thinkers may fault their negative attitudes for a poor recovery or job loss. Debbie Johnson, *Think Yourself Thin* (New York: Hyperion Books, 1996), back cover; Barbara Ehrenreich, "The Secret of Mass Delusion," *The Huffington Post*, February 27, 2007, http://www.huffingtonpost.com/barbara-ehrenreich/the-secret-of-mass-delusi_b_42212.html.

88 Jed Babbin, "Obama's Arugula Gap," *Human Events: Powerful Conservative Voices*, August 12, 2008, http://humanevents.com/2008/08/12/obamas-arugula-gap/.

89 Michael Pollan, "An Open Letter to the Next Farmer in Chief," *The New York Times Magazine*, October 12, 2008.

90 Centers for Disease Control and Prevention, "Obesity and Overweight," *National Center for Health Statistics*, http://www.cdc.gov/nchs/fastats/obesity-overweight.htm.

91 United States Department of Agriculture, *Growth Patterns in the U.S. Organic Industry*, October 2013, https://www.ers.usda.gov/amber-waves/2013/october/growth-patterns-in-the-us-organic-industry/.

92 Stephen Barrett, "Questionable Organizations: An Overview," *Quackwatch*, http://quackwatch.org/04ConsumerEducation/nonrecorg.html.

93 Woodson C. Merrell, *The Detox Prescription: Supercharge Your Health, Strip Away Pounds, and Eliminate the Toxins Within* (Emmaus, PA: Rodale Press), xvii.

94 Ibid., 170.

95 Ibid., 255.

96 Ibid., 10.

97 Silas Weir Mitchell counseled Charlotte Perkins Gilman as follows: "Lie down an hour after each meal. Have but two hours' intellectual life a day. And never touch pen, brush, or pencil as long as you live." Mitchell, qtd. in Anne Stiles, "The Rest Cure, 1873–1925," *BRANCH (Britain, Representation and Nineteenth-Century History)*, http://www.branchcollective.org/?ps_articles=anne-stiles-the-rest-cure-1873-1925.

98 Gail Bederman, *Manliness & Civilization: A Cultural History of Gender and Race in the United States, 1880–1917* (Chicago: University of Chicago Press, 1995), 131.

99 Merrell, *The Detox Prescription*, 67–68.

100 Ibid., 100–124.

CONCLUSION

1 Ralph Waldo Emerson, *Emerson in His Journals*, ed. Joel Porte (Cambridge, MA: Harvard University Press, 1982), 99.

2 Fedon Lindberg, *The GI Mediterranean Diet* (Berkeley, CA: Ulysses Press, 2009), 92; Robb Wolf, *The Paleo Solution: The Original Human Diet* (Las Vegas, NV: Victory Belt, 2010), 30; Valerie Alston, *Paleo Smoothies* (n.p.: Cooking Genius, 2014), 1.

3 George Malkmus, with Peter and Stowe Shockey, *The Hallelujah Diet: Experience the Optimal Health You Were Meant to Have* (Shippensburg, PA: Destiny Image Publishers, 2006), 46.

4 Terry Shintani, letter to author, July 25, 2014.

5 Angus Chen, "Diet Foods Are Tanking. So The Diet Industry Is Now Selling 'Health,'" *NPR*, January 26, 2016, http://www.npr.org/sections/thesalt/2016/01/20/462691546 /as-diet-foods-tank-confusing-health-labels-replace-them.

6 Patrick Rogers, "The Diet Is Dead," *Allure*, August 9, 2016, http://www.allure.com /story/calorie-counting-diet-trend-ending.

7 Khloé Kardashian, *Strong Looks Better Naked* (New York: Regan Arts, 2015), 86–89.

8 Deborah Brauser, "Orthorexia Nervosa: When 'Healthy' Eating Turns Dangerous," *Medscape*, May 31, 2017, http://www.medscape.com/viewarticle/880916#vp_2.

9 Esther Blum, *Cavewomen Don't Get Fat* (New York: Gallery Books, 2013), 20.

10 Helen Ayers Davis, *The New No Willpower Diet* (New York: McKay Co., 1970), 2. Emphasis in original.

11 Shelley Fisher Fishkin, *From Fact to Fiction: Journalism and Imaginative Writing in America* (New York: Oxford University Press, 1985), 5.

12 Guthman, *Weighing In*, 52.

13 Gwen E Chapman, "From 'Dieting' to 'Healthy Eating': An Exploration of Shifting Constructions of Eating for Weight Control," in *Interpreting Weight: The Social Management of Fatness and Thinness*, ed. Jeffrey Sobal and Donna Maurer (New York: Aldine de Gruyter, 1999), 85.

14 "Why Mindful Eating?," *The Center for Mindful Eating*, 2014, https://thecenterfor mindfuleating.org/Resources/Documents/TCME_2014_introbrochure.pdf.

15 Guthman, *Weighing In*, 52.

16 E. J. Schultz, "Lean Cuisine Makes 'Massive Pivot' Away from Diet Marketing," *Advertising Age*, June 26, 2015, http://adage.com/article/cmo-strategy/lean-cuisine-makes -massive-pivot-diet-marketing/299236/.

17 Roberto Ferdman, "The Chipotle Effect: Why America Is Obsessed with Fast Casual Food," *The Washington Post*, February 2, 2015.

18 Kate Taylor, "Chipotle's Stock Is Down after Claims of Food-Poisoning Incidents in Manhattan," *BusinessInsider*, July 7, 2016, http://www.businessinsider.com/chipotles -stock-down-after-reports-of-another-food-poisoning-2016-7.

19 Refers to both online and in-person subscribers on recurring billing plans. "Weight Watchers Announces First Quarter 2017 Results and Raises Full Year 2017 Guidance" (press release), *Weight Watchers International*, May 2017, http://www.weightwatchers international.com/file/Index?KeyFile=2000383267.

20 Ibid.

21 Morando Soffritti's study demonstrated that aspartame (the sweetener in Diet Coke) doubled cancer risk in rats. Though Soffritti's research was disputed by other scientists and the artificial sweetener industry, studies like his feed rumors about the dangers of artificial ingredients. Morando Soffritti, Fiorella Belpoggi, Eva Tibaldi, Davide

Degli Esposti, and Michelina Lauriola, "Life-Span Exposure to Low Doses of Aspartame Beginning during Prenatal Life Increases Cancer Effects in Rats," *Environmental Health Perspectives* 115, no. 9 (2007): 1293–1297.

22 Gyorgy Scrinis, "On the Ideology of Nutritionism," *Gastronomica* 8, no. 1 (2008): 39–48.

23 Jessica Mudry, *Measured Meals: Nutrition in America* (Albany: State University of New York Press, 2009), 36–39.

24 Rachel Laudan, *Cuisine and Empire: Cooking in World History* (Berkeley: University of California Press, 2013), 304.

25 Michael Pollan, "Six Rules for Eating Wisely," *Time*, June 11, 2006, 97.

26 So far, results have shown clinically significant weight loss, even after two years of implanted use. Six months after the approval of vBLOC, the FDA approved the Re-Shape Integrated Dual Balloon System, a temporary balloon that is inflated inside the stomach, creating feelings of satiety. Considered less innovative than vBloc, the balloon nonetheless offers a safer, less invasive alternative to the older gastric bands or stomach reduction surgeries. Food and Drug Administration, *EnteroMedics Maestro Rechargeable System—P130019*, January 16, 2015, https://www.fda.gov/MedicalDevices /ProductsandMedicalProcedures/DeviceApprovalsandClearances/Recently-Approved Devices/ucm430696.html.

27 Jonah Comstock, "7 Fitness Apps with 16 Million or More Downloads," *Mobi-HealthNews*, August 26, 2013, http://www.mobihealthnews.com/24958/7-fitness-apps -with-16-million-or-more-downloads/page/0/5.

28 Kat Stoeffel, "Created by Men, Women Now Playing Public Diet Game," *New York Magazine: The Cut*, April 25, 2013, https://www.thecut.com/2013/04/created-by-men-women-now-public-dieting.html.

29 Economists have found that salaries often rise when men join a female-dominant profession. Men still make substantially more than women, but men's entrance into the field will raise everyone's salary. A rising tide lifts all ships; men legitimate female-dominant fields—be it nursing, teaching, or dieting. Men like Jamie Oliver, Michael Pollan, and Loren Cordain have helped legitimate the food movement and, as the food movement began to be taken seriously, more and more men have joined.

30 Tim Ferris, *The 4-Hour Body: An Uncommon Guide to Rapid Fat-Loss, Incredible Sex, and Becoming Superhuman* (New York: Random House), 2010.

31 Tamar Adler, "When Meals Get Macho," *New Yorker*, October 26, 2012, http:// www.newyorker.com/culture/culture-desk/when-meals-get-macho.

32 Krishnendu Ray, "Domesticating Cuisine: Food and Aesthetics on American Television," *Gastronomica* 7, no. 1 (2007): 50–63.

33 Johnston and Baumann, *Foodies*.

34 United States Department of Agriculture, "USDA Reports Record Growth in U.S. Organic Producers" (press release), April 4, 2016, https://www.usda.gov/media/press -releases/2016/04/04/usda-reports-record-growth-us-organic-producers.

35 http://www.public.iastate.edu/~ethics/Prop2.pdf.

36 C. L. Ogden, M. D. Carroll, B. K. Kit, and K. M. Flegal, "Prevalence of Childhood and Adult Obesity in the United States, 2011–2012," *Journal of the American Medical Association* 311, no. 8 (2014): 806–814.

37 Martin Wabitsch, Anja Moss, and Katrin Kromeyer-Hauschild, "Unexpected Plateauing of Childhood Obesity Rates in Developed Countries," *BMC Public Health* 12, no. 17 (2014).

38 Clifford Geertz, "Deep Play: Notes on the Balinese Cockfight," in *The Interpretation of Cultures: Selected Essays* (New York: Basic Books, 1973), 448.

BIBLIOGRAPHY

Adams, Elvin. *Jesus Was Thin So You Can Be Thin Too*. Bloomington, IN: Universe, 2010.

Addison, Heather. *Hollywood and the Rise of Physical Culture*. New York: Routledge, 2003.

Adorno, Theodor. "The Culture Industry: Enlightenment as Mass Deception." In *The Dialectic of Enlightenment*, edited by Theodor Adorno and Max Horkheimer. New York: Continuum, 1995.

Aikau, Hokulani K. "Indigeneity in the Diaspora: The Case of Native Hawaiians at Iosepa, Utah." *American Quarterly* 62, no. 3 (2010): 477–500.

Albert-Matesz, Rachel, and Don Matesz. *The Garden of Eating: A Produce-Dominated Diet & Cookbook*. Phoenix, AZ: Planetary Press, 2004.

Allen, Carmel. "The 72-Hour Hangover Cure: Start a Detox Diet Today for a Clean Break before the New Year Binge." *Mail on Sunday*. December 27, 1998, 45.

Alston, Valerie. *Paleo Smoothies*. n.p. (eBook): Cooking Genius, 2014.

Aluli, Noa Emmett, Phillip W. Reyes, and JoAnn 'Umilani Tsark. "Cardiovascular Disease Disparities in Native Hawaiians." *Journal of the CardioMetabolic Syndrome* 2, no. 4 (Fall 2007): 250–253.

Ancestral Health Society. "Manifesto." *About AHS*. April 1, 2014, http://www.ancestral health.org/about.

Apple, Rima Dombrow. *Vitamania: Vitamins in American Culture*. New Brunswick, NJ: Rutgers University Press, 1996.

Audette, Ray, with Troy Gilchrist. *Neanderthin: Eat Like a Caveman to Achieve a Lean, Strong, Healthy Body*. New York: St. Martin's Press, 1999.

Babbin, Jed. "Obama's Arugula Gap." *Human Events: Powerful Conservative Voices*. August 12, 2008, http://humanevents.com/2008/08/12/obamas-arugula-gap/.

Baier, Leslie J., and Robert L. Hanson. "Genetic Studies of the Etiology of Type 2 Diabetes in Pima Indians: Hunting for Pieces to a Complicated Puzzle." *Diabetes* 53, no. 5 (2004): 1181–1186.

Bakhtin, Mikhail. *Rabelais and His World*. Cambridge, MA: MIT Press, 1968.

Barnard, Neal. *The 21-Day Weight Loss Kickstart*. New York: Grand Central Life & Style, 2011.

Barrett, Stephen. "Questionable Organizations: An Overview." *Quackwatch*. January 18, 2016, https://quackwatch.org/04ConsumerEducation/nonrecorg.html.

———. "Rev. George M. Malkmus and His Hallelujah Diet." *Quackwatch*. May 29, 2013, http://www.quackwatch.org/11Ind/malkmus.html.

Bederman, Gail. *Manliness & Civilization: A Cultural History of Gender and Race in the United States, 1880–1917*. Chicago: University of Chicago Press, 1995.

Belasco, Warren. *Appetite for Change: How the Counterculture Took On the Food Industry*. Ithaca, NY: Cornell University Press, 1989.

———. *Food: The Key Concepts*. New York: Berg, 2008.

Bennett, Oliver. *Cultural Pessimism: Narratives of Decline in the Postmodern World*. Edinburgh: Edinburgh University Press, 2001.

Bennett, P. H., T. A. Burch, and M. Miller. "Diabetes Mellitus in American (Pima) Indians." *The Lancet* 298, no. 7716 (July 17, 1971): 125–128.

Bentley, Amy. *Eating for Victory: Food Rationing and the Politics of Domesticity*. Chicago: University of Illinois Press, 1998.

Bercovitch, Sacvan. *The American Jeremiad*. Madison: University of Wisconsin Press, 1978.

Berger, Stuart. *Dr. Berger's Immune Power Diet*. New York: New American Library, 1985.

Biltekoff, Charlotte. *Eating Right in America: The Cultural Politics of Food and Health*. Durham, NC: Duke University Press, 2013.

Bingaman, Amy, Lise Sanders, and Rebecca Zorach. *Embodied Utopias: Gender, Social Change, and the Modern Metropolis*. London: Routledge, 2002.

Blackburn, George, and W. Allan Walker. "Science-Based Solutions to Obesity: What Are the Roles of Academia, Government, Industry, and Health Care?" *The American Journal of Clinical Nutrition* 82, no. 1 (July 1, 2005): 207–210.

Bloomgarden, Zachary. "International Diabetes Federation Meeting, 1997." *Diabetes Care* 21, no. 5 (May 1998): 860.

Blum, Esther. *Cavewomen Don't Get Fat*. New York: Gallery Books, 2013.

Blumenthal, Deborah. "A Day in the Life of the Betty Ford Center." *The New York Times*. February 27, 1987, 1.

Bordo, Susan. "Hunger as Ideology." In *Eating Culture*, edited by Ron Scapp and Brian Seitz. Albany: State University of New York Press, 1998.

———. *Unbearable Weight: Feminism, Western Culture, and the Body*. Berkeley: University of California Press, 2003.

Bourdieu, Pierre. *Masculine Domination*. Stanford, CA: Stanford University Press, 2001.

Bowman, Crystal, and Tricia Goyer. *Whit's End Mealtime Devotions: 90 Faith-Building Ideas Your Kids Will Eat Up!* Carol Stream, IL: Tyndale House, 2013.

Boyd Eaton, S., and Melvin Konner. "Paleolithic Nutrition—A Consideration of Its Nature and Current Implications." *New England Journal of Medicine* 312 (1985): 283–289.

Boyd Eaton, S., Melvin Konner, and Marjorie Shostak. "Stone Agers in the Fast Lane: Chronic Degenerative Diseases in Evolutionary Perspective." *The American Journal of Medicine* 84, no. 4 (1988).

Boym, Svetlana. *The Future of Nostalgia*. New York: Basic Books, 2001.

Bragg, Paul. *Healthful Eating without Confusion*. Desert Hot Springs, CA: Health Science, 1976.

Bragg, Paul, and Patricia Bragg. *The Miracle of Fasting Proven throughout History for Physical, Mental, & Spiritual Rejuvenation*. Santa Barbara, CA: Health Science, 1985.

Braziel, Jana Evans, and Kathleen LeBesco, eds. *Bodies out of Bounds: Fatness and Transgression*. Berkeley: University of California Press, 2001.

Brody, Jane. "Personal Health." *The New York Times*. December 25, 1996, C6.

Brown, Michael. "Can You Detox Your Body?" *American Health* 5 (1986): 53–58.

Brumberg, Joan Jacobs. *The Body Project: An Intimate History of American Girls*. New York: Random House, 1997.

———. "Fasting Girls: The Emerging Ideal of Slenderness in American Culture." In *Women's America: Refocusing the Past*, 8th ed., edited by Linda Kerber, Jane Sherron de Hart, Cornelia Hughes Dayton, and Judy Tzu-Chun Wu. New York: Oxford University Press, 2016.

Burlay, Anthony. *The Foundation Diet: Your Body Was Designed to Eat*. W. Hollywood, CA: Zen-Fusion Publishing, 2004.

Bynum, Caroline Walker. *Holy Feast and Holy Fast: The Religious Significance of Food to Medieval Women*. Berkeley: University of California Press, 1987.

Byrne, Rhonda. *The Secret*. New York: Atria Books, 2006.

Calbom, Cherie, and John Calbom. *The Coconut Diet*. New York: Warner Books, 2005.

Campbell, Hugh, Michael Bell, and Margaret Finney. *Country Boys: Masculinity and Rural Life*. University Park: Pennsylvania State University Press, 2006.

Campos, Paul. *The Obesity Myth: Why America's Obsession with Weight Is Hazardous to Your Health*. New York: Gotham Books, 2004.

Carpender, Dana. *500 Paleo Recipes: Hundreds of Delicious Recipes for Weight Loss and Super Health*. Beverly, MA: Fair Winds Press, 2012.

Carson, Rachel. *Silent Spring*. Boston: Houghton Mifflin, 1962.

Casid, Jill H. *Sowing Empire: Landscape and Colonization*. Minneapolis: University of Minnesota Press, 2005.

Cassell, Dana, and David Gleaves. "Religion and Obesity." In *The Encyclopedia of Obesity and Eating Disorders*, 258. New York: Infobase Publishing, 2006.

Cassels, Susan. "Overweight in the Pacific: Links between Foreign Dependence, Global Food Trade, and Obesity in the Federated States of Micronesia." *Globalization and Health* 2, no. 10 (2006).

Cavanaugh, Joan, and Pat Forseth. *More of Jesus, Less of Me*. Plainfield, NJ: Logos International, 1976.

Centers for Disease Control and Prevention. "Obesity and Overweight." *National Center for Health Statistics*. September 30, 2015, http://www.cdc.gov/nchs/fastats/obesity-over weight.htm.

Centers for Disease Control and Prevention, National Center for Health Statistics. *Health, United States, 2014: With Special Feature on Adults Aged 55–64*, 199. Hyattsville, MD: CDC, 2015.

Chapian, Maria, and Neva Coyle. *The All-New Free to Be Thin*. Minneapolis, MN: Bethany House, 1994.

———. *Free to Be Thin*. Minneapolis, MN: Bethany House, 1979.

Chapman, Gwen E. "From 'Dieting' to 'Healthy Eating': An Exploration of Shifting Constructions of Eating for Weight Control." In *Interpreting Weight: The Social Management of Fatness and Thinness*, edited by Jeffery Sobal and Donna Maurer, 73–87. New York: Aldine de Gruyter, 1999.

Clark, Constance Areson. "Evolution for John Doe: Pictures, the Public, and the Scopes Trial Debate." *Journal of American History* 87 (2001): 1275–1303.

———. *God—or Gorilla: Images of Evolution in the Jazz Age*. Baltimore: Johns Hopkins University Press, 2008.

Clarke, David. *Cinderella Meets the Caveman*. Eugene, OR: Harvest House Publishers, 2007.

Clifford, James. *Routes: Travel and Translation in the Late Twentieth Century*. Cambridge, MA: Harvard University Press, 1997.

Clifford, James, and George E. Marcus. *Writing Culture: The Poetics and Politics of Ethnography*. Berkeley: University of California Press, 1986.

Cohen, Jodie, and Gilaad Cohen. *The Everything Paleolithic Diet Book: An All-Natural, Easy-to-Follow Plan to Improve Health, Lose Weight, Increase Endurance, Prevent Disease*. Avon, MA: Adams Media, 2011.

Cohen, Roger. "Broken Men in Paradise." *The New York Times*. December 9, 2016.

Cole, Gene Wall. *Jesus' Diet for all the World*. Henrietta, NC: A.I. Publishing, 2005.

The Cook Book of Glorious Eating for Weight Watchers: Recipes and Menus from Wesson to Help Prevent Overweight. New Orleans, LA: Wesson People, 1961. In the Alan and Shirley Brocker Sliker Collection, MSS 314, Special Collections, Michigan State University Libraries.

Cordain, Loren. *The Paleo Answer: 7 Days to Lose Weight, Feel Great, Stay Young*. Hoboken, NJ: John Wiley & Sons, 2010.

———. *The Paleo Diet*. Hoboken, NJ: John Wiley & Sons, 2002.

———. *The Paleo Diet Cookbook*. Hoboken, NJ: John Wiley & Sons, 2011.

———. *The Real Paleo Diet Cookbook*. New York: Houghton Mifflin Harcourt, 2015.

Corkery, P. J. "Addiction à L.A. Mode." *New Republic*. July 7, 1985.

"Corpulence." *Scientific American* 47 (November 4, 1882): 289.

Costantini, Antonio, with H. Wieland and Lars I. Qvick. *The Garden of Eden Longevity Diet: Antifungal-Antimycotoxin Diet for the Prevention and Treatment of Cancer, Atherosclerosis (Coronary-Carotid Vascular Disease), and Other Degenerative Diseases*. Freiburg, Germany: Oberlin, 1998.

Counihan, Carole M., and Steven L. Kaplan. *Food and Gender: Identity and Power*. New York: Routledge, 1998.

Cox, Meki. "Hawaiians Find Better Health in Roots." *Los Angeles Times*. July 28, 2013.

Creed, James Jr. *Answers: As the Lightning Cometh Out of the East, and Shineth Even unto the West so Shall Also the Coming of the Son of Man Be*. Bloomington, IN: Xlibris Corporation, 2003.

Crews, Douglas, and Barry Bogin. "Growth, Development, Senescence, and Aging: A Life History Perspective." In *A Companion to Biological Anthropology*, edited by Clark Spencer Larsen. Oxford: Wiley-Blackwell, 2010.

Cubbison Cracker Company. *Cubbison's Party Guide: Slenderizing Menus and Recipes*. Los Angeles: Cubbison Cracker Co., 1933.

Curtis, Michael. "The Obesity Epidemic in the Pacific." *Journal of Development and Social Transformation* 1: 37–42.

D'Adamo, Peter, and Catherine Whitney. *Eat Right 4 Your Type: The Individualized Blood Type Diet Solution*. New York: Berkley Press, 2016.

———. *Eat Right 4 Your Type: The Individualized Diet Solution to Staying Healthy, Living Longer, and Achieving Your Ideal Weight*. New York: G. P. Putnam's Sons, 1996.

Dalrymple, Theodore. "A Lesson from the Pacific." *New Statesman* 15, no. 724 (September 2002): 16.

D'Angelo, Charles. *Think and Grow Thin*. Mississauga, ON: Robert Kennedy Publishing, 2012.

"Dangers in Diets." Review of *Diet and Die* by Carl Malmberg. *The New York Times*. October 13, 1935, BR12.

"Dangers of the Diet Fad." *Yorkville Enquirer* (South Carolina). February 24, 1897. In *Chronicling America: Historic American Newspapers* (Library of Congress), http://chronicling america.loc.gov/.

Daniels, Mary. "Gloria Urges, Quit Taking Your Lumps of Sugar." *Chicago Tribune*. April 11, 1976.

Dart, J. "Book Pits Faith against Fat." *Los Angeles Times*. July 10, 1976.

Davis, Carole, and Etta Saltos. "Dietary Recommendations and How They Have Changed over Time." In *America's Eating Habits: Changes and Consequences*, edited by E. Frazao, 35. Washington, DC: United States Department of Agriculture, 1999.

Davis, Helen Ayers. *The New No Willpower Diet without Cyclamates*. New York: McKay, 1970.

Davis, Kara. *Spiritual Secrets to Weight Loss*. Lake Mary, FL: Charisma Media, 2002.

de Groot, Roy. *How I Reduced with the New Rockefeller Diet*. New York: Horizon Press, 1956.

de la Peña, Carolyn. *Empty Pleasures: The Story of Artificial Sweeteners from Saccharin to Splenda*. Chapel Hill: University of North Carolina Press, 2010.

Deloria, Philip. *Playing Indian*. New Haven, CT: Yale University Press, 1998.

DeLuz, Roni. *21 Pounds in 21 Days: The Martha's Vineyard Diet Detox*. New York: Harper Collins, 2007.

D'Emilio, John, and Estelle Freedman. *Intimate Matters: A History of Sexuality in America*. New York: Harper & Row, 1988.

Denoon, Donald, with Stewart Firth, Jocelyn Linnekin, Malama Meleisea, and Karen Nero. *The Cambridge History of the Pacific Islanders*. Cambridge: Cambridge University Press, 1997.

Densmore, Emmet. *The Natural Food of Man: A Brief Statement of the Principal Arguments against the Use of Bread, Cereals, Pulses, and All Other Starch Foods*. London: Pewtress and Co., 1890.

"Detox Diet Is Key to a Sizzling Summer." *The Mirror*. June 29, 1999, 20.

de Vany, Arthur. *The New Evolution Diet: What Our Paleolithic Ancestors Can Teach Us about Weight Loss, Fitness, and Aging*. Emmaus, PA: Rodale Press, 2010.

de Villiers, Jean-Pierre. *77 Ways to Reshape Your Life*. Herts, AL: Ecademy Press, 2011.

Diner, Hasia. *Hungering for America: Italian, Irish, and Jewish Foodways in the Age of Migration*. Cambridge, MA: Harvard University Press, 2001.

Dorfman, Lisa. *The Tropical Diet: A Scientific, Simple, & Sexy Weight Loss Strategy*. Miami, FL: Food Fitness International, 2004.

Douglas, Bernadine, and Bridgette Allan. *The Banting Solution: Your Low-Carb Guide to Permanent Weight Loss*. Cape Town, South Africa: Penguin, 2016.

Dufty, William. *Sugar Blues*. Radnor, PA: Chilton Book Company, 1975.

Dumke, Edward. *The Serpent Beguiled Me and I Ate: A Heavenly Diet for Saints and Sinners*. Garden City, NY: Doubleday, 1986.

DuPuis, E. Melanie. *Dangerous Digestion: The Politics of American Dietary Advice*. Berkeley: University of California Press, 2015.

Durant, John. *The Paleo Manifesto: Ancient Wisdom for Lifelong Health*. New York: Random House, 2013.

Dworkin, Norine. "Seasonal Detox: Supercharge Your Health with a Personal Purification Program." *Vegetarian Times*, March 1999, 46.

Dworkin, Shari, and Faye Wachs. *Body Panic: Gender, Health, and the Selling of Fitness*. New York: New York University Press, 2009.

Dye, Tom. "Population Trends in Hawaii before 1778." *Hawaiian Journal of History* (1994): 1–20.

"Eat and Remain Young, French Secret for Beauty." *The Washington Post*. January 15, 1911.

Edwards, Darryl, with Brett Stewart and Jason Warner. *Paleo Fitness*. Berkeley, CA: Ulysses Press, 2013.

Egan, Hope. "Rewire Your Taste Buds—Can You Give God Your Appetite?" *Faith and Fitness Magazine*. December 2009, http://faithandfitness.net/node/2818.

Ehrenreich, Barbara. "The Secret of Mass Delusion." *Huffington Post*. February 27, 2007, http://www.huffingtonpost.com/barbara-ehrenreich/the-secret-of-mass-delusi_b_42212.html.

Elias, Megan J. *Food in the United States, 1890–1945*. Santa Barbara, CA: Greenwood Press, 2009.

Ellin, Abby. "Flush Those Toxins! Eh, Not So Fast." *The New York Times*. January 7, 2014.

Ellison, Christopher, and Jeffrey Levin. "The Religion-Health Connection: Evidence, Theory, and Future Directions." *Health Education and Behavior* 25, no. 6 (1998): 700–720.

Federal Trade Commission. "Dietary Supplement Maker Garden of Life Settles FTC Charges" (press release). March 9, 2006, https://www.ftc.gov/news-events/press-releases/2006/03/dietary-supplement-maker-garden-life-settles-ftc-charges.

Fekner, John. "Toxic Junkie Text Entry." *Research Archive*. 2010, http://johnfekner.com/feknerArchive/?p=1249#more-1249.

Ferreira, Mariana K. Leal, and Gretchen Chesley Lang. *Indigenous Peoples and Diabetes: Community Empowerment and Wellness*. Durham, NC: Carolina Academic Press, 2006.

Fertig, David. *Analogy and Morphological Change*. Edinburgh: Edinburgh University Press, 2013.

Fields, Leslie Leyland. "The Fitness-Driven Church." *Christianity Today*. June 21, 2013, http://www.christianitytoday.com/ct/2013/june/fitness-driven-church.html.

Finn, Stephanie Mariko. "Aspirational Eating: Class Anxiety and the Rise of Food in Popular Culture." PhD diss., University of Michigan, 2011.

Fishkin, Shelley Fisher. *From Fact to Fiction: Journalism and Imaginative Writing in America*. New York: Oxford University Press, 1985.

Fitzpatrick-Nietschmann, Judith. "Pacific Islanders—Migration and Health." *Western Journal of Medicine* 139, no. 6 (December 1983): 848–853.

Floresca, Jeanne. *Paleo Traveler: Old World Recipes Flipped NeoPaleo*. n.p. (eBook): Bookbaby, 2014.

Fogarty, Robert S. "An Imaginary Country" (editorial). *The Antioch Review* 63, no. 4 (Autumn 2005): 613–614.

Foliaki, Sonia, and Neil Pearce. "Prevalence and Causes of Diabetes in Pacific Populations." *Pacific Health Dialog* 10, no. 2 (2003): 90.

Foucault, Michel. "On the Genealogy of Ethics: An Overview of a Work in Progress." In *Michel Foucault: Beyond Structuralism and Hermeneutics*, edited by Hubert Dreyfus and Paul Rabinow. Chicago: University of Chicago Press, 1983.

Foxcroft, Louise. *Calories and Corsets: A History of Dieting over Two Thousand Years*. London: Profile Books, 2011.

Fredericks, Kate. *What Is Paleo Diet?* n.p. (eBook): CreateSpace Independent Publishing Platform, 2012.

Freudenheim, Milt. "Employers Focus on Weight as Workplace Health Issue: Medical Costs Rising as Nation Gets Heavier." *The New York Times*. September 6, 1999.

Fromson, Daniel. "The New Yorker Weighs In on the Foodie Elitism Debate." *The Atlantic*. July 15, 2010, www.theatlantic.com/health/archive/2010/07/the-new-yorker-weighs-in-on-the-foodie-elitism-debate/59815/.

Furnas, J. C. *Anatomy of Paradise: Hawaii and the Islands of the South Seas*. New York: William Sloane Associates, 1948.

Gabriel, Jon. *Visualization for Weight Loss: The Gabriel Method Guide to Using Your Mind to Transform Your Body*. Carlsbad, CA: Hay House, 2015.

Garland-Thomson, Rosemarie. *Extraordinary Bodies: Figuring Physical Disability in American Culture and Literature*. New York: Columbia University Press, 1997.

Garrett, Brenda. "England, Colonialism, and 'The Land of Cokaygne.'" *Utopian Studies* 15, no. 1 (2004): 1–12.

Garth, Jennifer. *Adam and Eve Weren't Fat*. Milsons Point, NSW: Random House Australia, 1999.

Gatehouse, Judy. "Home." *Hungry for Jesus*." 2016, http://www.hungryforjesus.org/.

Gerber, Lynne. "Fat Christians and Fit Elites: Negotiating Class and Status in Evangelical Christian Weight-Loss Culture." *American Quarterly* 64, no. 1 (March 2012).

Gewertz, Deborah B., and Frederick Karl Errington. *Cheap Meat: Flap Food Nations in the Pacific Islands*. Berkeley: University of California Press, 2010.

Giddens, Anthony. *Modernity and Self-Identity: Self and Society in the Late Modern Age*. Stanford, CA: Stanford University Press, 1991.

Gilman, Sander. *Diets and Dieting: A Cultural Encyclopedia*. New York: Routledge, 2008.

———. *Obesity: The Biography*. Oxford: Oxford University Press, 2010.

Goldfarb, Robert S., Thomas C. Leonard, and Steven Suranovic. "Modeling Alternative Motives for Dieting." *Eastern Economic Journal* 32, no. 1 (Winter 2006).

Goode, Sam. *Why You Should Not Have Sex before Marriage: The Christian Perspective*. Norwalk, CA: Hermit Kingdom Press, 2006.

Graham, Sylvester. *Lectures on the Science of Human Life*. Boston: Marsh, Capen, Lyon, and Webb, 1839.

———. *A Lecture to Young Men on Chastity*. Boston: Light & Stearns, Crocker & Brewster, 1837.

Gregory, James. *Of Victorians and Vegetarians: The Vegetarian Movement in Nineteenth-Century Britain*. London: Tauris Academic Studies, 2007.

Griffith, R. Marie. *Born Again Bodies: Flesh and Spirit in American Christianity*. Berkeley: University of California Press, 2004.

———. "'Don't Eat That': The Erotics of Abstinence in American Christianity." *Gastronomica: The Journal of Food and Culture* 1, no. 4 (Fall 2001): 36–47.

Guha, Ranajit, and Gayatri Chakravorty Spivak. *Selected Subaltern Studies*. New York: Oxford University Press, 1988.

Guthman, Julie. *Weighing In: Obesity, Food Justice, and the Limits of Capitalism*. Berkeley: University of California Press, 2011.

Haas, Elson. *The Detox Diet: A How and When-to Guide for Cleansing the Body*. Berkeley, CA: Celestial Arts, 1996.

Haas, Elson, and Cameron Stauth. *The False Fat Diet: The Revolutionary 21-Day Program for Losing the Weight You Think Is Fat*. New York: Ballantine Books, 2001.

Haber, Barbara. *From Hardtack to Homefries: An Uncommon History of American Cooks and Meals*. New York: Free Press, 2002.

Haggard, Ted. *The Jerusalem Diet: The "One Day" Approach to Reach Your Ideal Weight—and Stay There*. Colorado Springs, CO: Waterbrook Press, 2005.

Halliday, Arthur, and Judy Wardell Halliday. *Get Thin, Stay Thin: A Biblical Approach to Food, Eating, and Weight Management*. Grand Rapids, MI: Revell Books, 2007.

Halstead, Pauli. *Primal Cuisine*. Rochester, VT: Healing Arts Press, 2012.

Hancock, Rita. *The Eden Diet: You Can Eat Treats, Enjoy Your Food, and Lose Weight*. Grand Rapids, MI: Zondervan, 2010.

Handler, Richard, and Jocelyn Linnekin. "Tradition, Genuine or Spurious." *Journal of American Folklore* 97, no. 385 (September 1984): 273–290.

Hanley, Charles. "Pacific Islanders Top the Scales." *Charleston Gazette*. May 10, 2004.

Hardin, Jessica, and Christina Kwauk. "Producing Markets, Producing People: Local Food, Financial Prosperity and Health in Samoa." *Food, Culture, and Society* 18, no. 3: 519–539.

Harrell, Jennie. "Is Paleo Expensive?" (blog). *EasyPaleo*. January 28, 2012, http://www.easypaleo.com/is-paleo-expensive-my-thoughts-money-saving-tips/.

Hawaii Department of Health. "Obesity in Hawaii Rising alongside National Trends" (press release). *Healthy Hawai'i Initiative*. August 21, 2013, http://health.hawaii.gov/news/files/2013/05/13-047-Press-Release-F-as-in-Fat.pdf.

"Hawaiian Race Vanishing, Says U.S. Naturalist." *San Francisco Chronicle*. April 11, 1920.

Hayenga, Elizabeth Sharon. "Dieting through the Decades: A Comparative Study of Weight Reduction in America as Depicted in Popular Literature and Books from 1940 to the late 1980s." PhD diss., University of Minnesota, 1989.

Hazelwood, Dan. "Rising Tide of Diabetes among Pacific Islanders" (podcast transcript). *Centers for Disease Control and Prevention*. May 2008, https://www2c.cdc.gov/podcasts/media/pdf/RisingTidePI.pdf.

Henn, Debra, and Deborah DeEugenio. *Diet Pills*. Philadelphia: Chelsea House, 2005.

Hershoff, Asa. *Homeopathic Remedies: A Quick and Easy Guide to Common Disorders and Their Homeopathic Treatments*. Garden City Park, NY: Avery Publishing Group, 1999.

Hesse-Biber, Sharlene. *The Cult of Thinness.* New York: Oxford University Press, 2007.

Hill, Sarah. *Paleo Diet.* n.p. (eBook): MaxHouse, 2013.

Hobsbawm, Eric, and Terence Ranger, eds. *The Invention of Tradition.* Cambridge: Cambridge University Press, 1983.

Hofmekler, Ori, and Diana Holtzberg. *The Warrior Diet.* St. Paul, MN: Dragon Door Publications, 2001.

Hofve, Jean, and Celeste Yarnall. *Paleo Dog: Give Your Best Friend a Long Life, Healthy Weight, and Freedom from Illness by Nurturing His Inner Wolf.* Emmaus, PA: Rodale Press, 2014.

"Holds Missionaries Degrade Pagan Races." *The New York Times.* February 20, 1926.

Horne, Charles Francis, and Julius August Brewer. *The Bible and Its Story: Taught by One Thousand Picture Lessons.* New York: F. R. Niglutsch, 1908.

Horsman, Reginald. *The New Republic: The United States of America 1789-1815.* New York: Routledge, 2000.

Hoverd, William James. *Working Out My Salvation: The Contemporary Gym and the Promise of "Self" Transformation.* Oxford: Meyer & Meyer Sport, 2005.

Huckabee, Mike. *Quit Digging Your Grave with a Knife and Fork: A 12-Stop Program to End Bad Habits and Begin a Healthy Lifestyle.* New York: Center Street, 2005.

Hughes, Claire Ku'uleilani. "E ala! E alu! E kuilima!—Up! Together! Join hands!" *Ka Wai Ola* 29, no. 3 (March/Malaki 2012): 20.

Hughes, Robert George. *Diet, Food Supply, and Obesity in the Pacific.* Manila, Philippines: World Health Organization, Regional Office for the Western Pacific, 2003.

Hurst, Fannie. *No Food with My Meals.* New York: Harper & Brothers, 1935.

Hussain, Shafqat. *Remoteness and Modernity: Transformation and Continuity in Northern Pakistan.* New Haven, CT: Yale University Press, 2015.

Hyman, Mark. *The Blood Sugar Solution 10-Day Detox Diet: Activate Your Body's Natural Ability to Burn Fat and Lose Weight Fast.* New York: Little, Brown, 2014.

Iacobbo, Karen, and Michael Iacobbo. *Vegetarian America: A History.* Westport, CT: Prager, 2004.

Inglis, Pat. "Gloria Swanson Talks of Food, Not Films." *The Montreal Gazette.* August 23, 1977.

Innanen, Summer. "Breaking the Diet-Sabotage Cycle." Poster and program at the Ancestral Health Society Symposium, Berkeley, CA, August 2014.

Jackson, Mark. *Allergy: The History of a Modern Malady.* London: Reaktion, 2006.

James, Ursula. *You Can Think Yourself Thin: Transform Your Shape with Hypnosis.* New York: Jeremy P. Tarcher/Penguin, 2009.

Jamieson, Alex. *The Great American Detox Diet: 8 Weeks to Weight Loss and Well-Being.* Emmaus, PA: Rodale Press, 2005.

Jaminet, Paul, and Shou-Ching Jaminet. *Perfect Health Diet: Regain Health and Lose Weight by Eating the Way You Were Meant to Eat.* New York: Scribner, 2012.

Jantz, Gregory. *The Spiritual Path to Weight Loss: Praising God by Living a Healthy Life.* Lincolnwood, IL: Publications International, 2000.

Johnson, Debbie. *Think Yourself Thin.* New York: Hyperion Books, 1996.

Johnston, Josée, and Shyon Baumann, *Foodies: Democracy and Distinction in the Gourmet Foodscape.* New York: Routledge, 2015.

Jolliffe, Norman. *Reduce and Stay Reduced*. New York: Simon and Schuster, 1952.

Jou, Chin. "The Biology and Genetics of Obesity—A Century of Inquiries." *New England Journal of Medicine* 2014, no. 370 (May 15, 2014): 1874–1877.

Joulwan, Melissa, and Kellyann Petrucci. *Living Paleo for Dummies*. Hoboken, NJ: John Wiley & Sons, 2013.

Kain, Ida Jean. "Maybe Your Appestat Needs Reconditioning." *The Washington Post*. August 27, 1952.

Kapur, Cari Costanzo. "Rights, Roots, and Resistance: Land and Indigenous (trans)Nationalism in Contemporary Hawai'i." PhD diss., Stanford University, 2005.

Kardashian, Khloé. *Strong Looks Better Naked*. New York: Regan Arts, 2015.

Keating, Joshua. "Why Do the World's Fattest People Live on Islands?" *Foreign Policy*. February 9, 2011, http://foreignpolicy.com/2011/02/09/why-do-the-worlds-fattest-people-live-on-islands/.

Keep Slim and Trim with Domino Sugar Menus. New York: American Sugar Refining Co., 1954. In the Alan and Shirley Brocker Sliker Collection, MSS 314, Special Collections, Michigan State University Libraries.

Keeping Your Weight Down! The Welch Way to Weight Control. New York: The Welch Grape Juice Co., 1933. In the Alan and Shirley Brocker Sliker Collection, MSS 314, Special Collections, Michigan State University Libraries.

Kēhaulani Kauanui, J. *Hawaiian Blood: Colonialism and the Politics of Sovereignty and Indigeneity*. Durham, NC: Duke University Press, 2008.

Kellogg, John Harvey. *The Battle Creek Sanitarium System: History, Organization, Methods*. Battle Creek, MI: Gage Printing, 1908.

———. *The Natural Diet of Man*. Battle Creek, MI: Modern Medicine Publishing Company, 1923.

Kemp, Melody. "Extinction in a Bottle." *Global Times*. May 20, 2013.

Kim, Jean. "Experimental Encounters: Filipino and Hawaiian Bodies in the U.S. Imperial Invention of Odontoclasia." *American Quarterly* 63, no. 2 (September 2010): 523–546.

Kim, K. H., with J. Sobal and E. Wethington. "Religion and Body Weight." *International Journal of Obesity and Related Metabolic Disorders* 4 (April 27, 2003): 469–477.

Kimmel, Michael. *The History of Men: Essays in the History of American and British Masculinities*. New York: State University of New York Press, 2005.

"Kitty Dukakis Admits Addiction to Diet Pills for 26 Years." *Orlando Sentinel*. July 9, 1987, A4.

Kopp, James. "Cosimo Noto's The Ideal City 1903: New Orleans as Medical Utopia." *Utopian Studies* 1, no. 2 (1990): 115–122.

Kresser, Chris. *Your Personal Paleo Code: The 3-Step Plan to Lose Weight, Reverse Disease, and Stay Fit and Healthy for Life*. New York: Little, Brown, 2013.

Kupfer, Charles. "Il Duce and the Father of Physical Culture." *Iron Game History* 6, no. 2 (January 2000): 3–9.

Kuska, Bob. "Breast Cancer Increases on Papua New Guinea." *Journal of the National Cancer Institute* 91, no. 12 (1999): 994–996.

La Forte, Jennifer. "Internal Cleansing & Detoxification." *Yoga Journal.* January–February 1997, 93.

Lal, Brij V., and Kate Fortune, eds. "Fatal Impact." In *The Pacific Islands: An Encyclopedia.* Honolulu: University of Hawaii Press, 2000.

Laudan, Rachel. *Cuisine and Empire: Cooking in World History.* Berkeley: University of California Press, 2013.

———. *The Food of Paradise: Exploring Hawaii's Culinary Heritage.* Honolulu: University of Hawaii Press, 1996.

"Lauds Caveman's Diet." *Chicago Defender.* March 27, 1926.

Levenstein, Harvey. *Fear of Food: A History of Why We Worry about What We Eat.* Chicago: University of Chicago Press, 2012.

Levine, Deborah. "Corpulence and Correspondence: President William H. Taft and the Medical Management of Obesity." *Annals of Internal Medicine* 159 (2013): 565–570.

Levitas, Ruth. *The Concept of Utopia.* London: Philip Allan, 1990.

———. "Educated Hope: Ernst Bloch on Abstract and Concrete Utopia." *Utopian Studies* 1, no. 2 (1990): 18.

Lewis, George. "From Minnesota Fat to Seoul Food: Spam in America and the Pacific Rim." *The Journal of Popular Culture* 34, no. 2 (Fall 2000): 83–105.

Lewis, R.W.B. *The American Adam: Innocence, Tragedy, and Tradition in the Nineteenth Century.* Chicago: University of Chicago Press, 1955.

Liburd, Leandris. *Diabetes and Health Disparities: Community-Based Approaches for Racial and Ethnic Populations.* New York: Springer, 2010.

Lindberg, Fedon. *The GI Mediterranean Diet: The Glycemic Index-Based Life-Saving Diet of the Greeks.* Berkeley, CA: Ulysses Press, 2009.

Liponis, Mark. *The Hunter/Farmer Diet Solution.* Carlsbad, CA: Hay House, 2012.

Lovett, C. S. *Help Lord—The Devil Wants Me Fat!* Baldwin Park, CA: Personal Christianity, 1977.

Lyons, Paul. *American Pacificism: Oceania in the U.S. Imagination.* New York: Routledge, 2006.

———. "From Man-Eaters to Spam-Eaters: Literary Tourism and the Discourse of Cannibalism from Herman Melville to Paul Theroux." In *Multiculturalism and Representation: Selected Essays,* edited by John Rieder and Larry E. Smith. Honolulu: University of Hawaii Press, 1996.

Macdonald, Barrie. "'Now an Island Is Too Big': Limits and Limitations of Pacific Islands History." *Journal of Pacific Studies* 20 (1996): 20–27.

Madden, Etta, and Martha L. Finch. *Eating in Eden: Food and American Utopias.* Lincoln: University of Nebraska Press, 2006.

Madsen, Deborah. *The Routledge Companion to Native American Literature.* New York: Routledge, 2015.

Malkmus, George, with Peter and Stowe Shockey. *The Hallelujah Diet: Experience the Optimal Health You Were Meant to Have.* Shippensburg, PA: Destiny Image Publishers, 2006.

Mankovitz, Roy. *The Original Diet: The Omnivore's Solution Designed by Nature, Researched by a Rocket Scientist.* Santa Barbara, CA: Montecito Wellness, 2008.

Manton, Catherine. *Fed Up: Women and Food in America.* Westport, CT: Bergin & Garvey, 1999.

Margolis, Marc. "Paying for a Chance to Suffer in Silence." *Newsweek.* May 26, 2008.

Marin, Louis. *Food for Thought.* Baltimore: Johns Hopkins University Press, 1989.

Markel, Howard. "John Harvey Kellogg and the Pursuit of Wellness." *Journal of the American Medical Association* 305, no. 17 (2011): 1814–1815.

Marketdata Enterprises. *The U.S. Weight Loss Market: 2014 Status Report & Forecast.* February 20, 2014, https://www.marketdataenterprises.com/wp-content/uploads/2014/01/Diet -Market-2014-Status-Report.pdf.

Marx, Karl. *Capital,* vol. 1. London: Penguin Classics, 1990.

Massas, Tyler. "Paleo and Low-Carb Living" (blog). *PaleoTyler.* http://www.paleotyler.com /paleo-comics.html.

McAnnaly, Brian. *Life after Death & Heaven and Hell.* Cape Town, South Africa: Struik Christian Books, 2009.

McCarthy, Laura Flynn. "Born Losers: The New Diet Junkies." *Mademoiselle: The Magazine for the Smart Young Woman* 94 (March 1988): 156, 232–233.

McCarrison, Robert. "The Nation's Larder in Wartime: Medical Aspects of the Use of Food." *The British Medical Journal* 1, no. 4145 (1940): 984–987.

———. *Studies in Deficiency Disease.* London: Henry Frowde and Hodder & Stoughton, 1921.

McCaughey, Martha. *The Caveman Mystique: Pop-Darwinism and the Debates over Sex, Violence, and Science.* New York: Routledge, 2008.

McDermott, Robyn. "Ethics, Epidemiology and the Thrifty Gene: Biological Determinism as a Health Hazard." *Social Science & Medicine* 47, no. 9 (November 1998): 1189–1195.

McGarvey, S. T. "Obesity in Samoans and a Perspective on Its Etiology in Polynesians." *American Journal of Critical Nutrition* 53, no. 6 (June 1991): 1586–1594.

McNeil, Legs. "Yuppie Like Me," *Spin* 4, no. 9 (1988): 92–95, 118.

Mein, Carolyn. *Different Bodies, Different Diets: Discover a Health and Diet Plan That Fits You.* New York: Regan Books, 2001.

Meister, Kathleen, and Marjorie Doyle. *Obesity and Food Technology.* New York: American Council on Science and Health, 2009.

Melville, Herman. *Typee: A Peep at Polynesian Life,* edited by Harrison Hayford, Hershel Parker, and G. Thomas Tanselle. Chicago: Northwestern University Press, 1968.

Merrell, Woodson. *The Detox Prescription: Supercharge Your Health, Strip Away Pounds, and Eliminate the Toxins Within.* Emmaus, PA: Rodale Press, 2013.

Meyer, Joyce. *Look Great, Feel Great: 12 Keys to Enjoying a Healthy Life Now.* New York: Warner Faith, 2006.

Miller, Daphne, and Allison Sarubin-Fragakis. *The Jungle Effect: A Doctor Discovers the Healthiest Diets from around the World,* 52–56 (Kauila Clark). New York: Collins, 2008.

Miller, Donald. *Easy Health Diet: Manage Weight and Prevent Scary Diseases.* Salt Lake City, UT: Thimk.Biz, 2004.

Miller, Perry. *The New England Mind: From Colony to Province*. Cambridge, MA: Harvard University Press, 1953.

Mitchell, W.J.T. *Landscape and Power*. Chicago: University of Chicago Press, 1994.

Moalem, Sharon. *The DNA Restart: Unlock Your Personal Genetic Code to Eat for Your Genes, Lose Weight, and Reverse Aging*. Emmaus, PA: Rodale Press, 2016.

Mollen, Art. *The Mollen Method: A 30-Day Program to Lifetime Health Addiction*. Emmaus, PA: Rodale Press, 1986.

Monaghan, Lee F. *Men and the War on Obesity: A Sociological Study*. London: Routledge, 2008.

Mudry, Jessica. *Measured Meals: Nutrition in America*. Albany: State University of New York Press, 2009.

Munro, Doug, and Brij V. Lal. *Texts and Contexts: Reflections in Pacific Islands Historiography*. Honolulu: University of Hawaii Press, 2006.

Nabhan, Gary Paul. *Why Some Like It Hot: Food, Genes, and Cultural Diversity*. Washington, DC: Island Press/Shearwater Books, 2004.

Nash, Linda. "Finishing Nature: Harmonizing Bodies and Environments in Late-Nineteenth-Century California." *Environmental History* 8, no. 1 (January 2003): 25–52.

National Institute of Diabetes and Digestive Kidney Diseases. *Overweight and Obesity Statistics*. October 2012, https://www.niddk.nih.gov/health-information/health-statistics/overweight-obesity.

Nickerson, Jane. "News of Food: City Nutrition Expert Explains in Book How to Reduce and Stay at Right Weight." *The New York Times*. May 20, 1952, 28.

Nienhiser, Jill. "About the Foundation." *The Weston A. Price Foundation*. http://www.westonaprice.org/about-us/about-the-foundation/.

Nietzsche, Friedrich. *The Use and Abuse of History*, trans. Adrian Collins. Indianapolis, IN: Bobbs-Merrill, 1957.

Nishiyama, Takaaki. "Nauru: An Island Plagued by Obesity and Diabetes." *The Asahi Shimbun Globe*. May 27, 2012.

O'Gorman, Patricia. *The Girly Thoughts 10-Day Detox Plan: The Resilient Woman's Guide to Saying No to Negative Self-Talk and Yes to Personal Power*. Deerfield Beach, FL: Health Communications, 2014.

Oliver, Douglas. *The Pacific Islands*. Cambridge, MA: Harvard University Press, 1951.

Omartian, Stormie. *Greater Health, God's Way: Seven Steps to Health, Youthfulness and Vitality*. Canoga Park, CA: Sparrow Press, 1984.

Opie, John. *Nature's Nation: An Environmental History of the United States*. Fort Worth, TX: Harcourt, 1998.

Orbach, Susie. *Fat Is a Feminist Issue: The Anti-Diet Guide to Permanent Weight Loss*. New York: Paddington Press, 1978.

Ortigara Crego, Lisa. "The Experience of a Spiritual Recovery from Food Addiction: A Heuristic Inquiry." PhD diss., Capella University, 2006.

Paleo Foundation. "Our Mission." *Paleo Foundation*. March 11, 2014, http://paleofoundation.org/about-us/.

Paradis, Elise. "Changing Meanings of Fat: Fat, Obesity, Epidemics, and America's Children." PhD diss., Stanford University, 2011.

Patenaud, Bertrand M. *A Wealth of Ideas: Revelations from the Hoover Institution Archives.* Stanford, CA: Stanford General Books, 2006.

Peters, Lulu Hunt. *Diet and Health, with Key to the Calories.* Chicago: The Reilly and Lee Co., 1918.

Pettegrew, John. *Brutes in Suits: Male Sensibility in America, 1890–1920.* Baltimore: Johns Hopkins University Press, 2007.

Pierce, Deborah, as told to Frances Spatz Leighton. "I Prayed Myself Slim." *The Washington Post.* April 10, 1960.

"The Pink Bread Fad: The Color of Foods Believed to Be Indicative of Personal Character and Are Easily Arranged." *Los Angeles Times.* November 9, 1913.

Pitts, Victoria. *In the Flesh: The Cultural Politics of Body Modification.* New York: Palgrave Macmillan, 2003.

Pollack, Herbert. "Reduce and Stay Reduced." *American Journal of Public Health and the Nation's Health* 42, no. 11 (1952): 1482–1483.

Pollan, Michael. *The Omnivore's Dilemma: A Natural History of Four Meals.* New York: Penguin, 2006.

———. "An Open Letter to the Next Farmer in Chief." *The New York Times Magazine.* October 12, 2008.

———. "Six Rules for Eating Wisely." *Time.* June 11, 2006.

Porterfield, Amanda. *Female Piety in Puritan New England: The Emergence of Religious Humanism.* New York: Oxford University Press, 1992.

Pratt, Steven. "Far-Flung Flavors: Looking for the Future of Hawaii's Food in Its Past." *Chicago Tribune.* August 26, 2003.

Price, Weston. *Nutrition and Physical Degeneration: A Comparison of Primitive and Modern Diets and Their Effects, etc.* New York: P. B. Hoeber, 1939.

Quillin, Martha. "Eats of Eden." *McClatchy-Tribune Business News.* December 10, 2006, 1.

Randolph, Theron. "The Descriptive Features of Food Addiction: Addictive Eating and Drinking." *Quarterly Journal of Studies on Alcohol* 17, no. 2 (1956): 198–224.

Randolph, Theron, and Ralph Moss. *An Alternative Approach to Allergies: How the New Field of Clinical Ecology Unravels the Environmental Causes of Mental and Physical Ills.* New York: Bantam Books, 1982.

Rasmussen, Nicolas. *On Speed: The Many Lives of Amphetamine.* New York: New York University Press, 2008.

Recchi, Ray. "Semantic Shenanigans as Low as You Can Go." *Sun Sentinel* (Florida). March 27, 1989.

Regan, Amanda. *"Madame Sylvia of Hollywood and Physical Culture, 1920–1940."* MA thesis, California State University San Marcos, 2013.

Reischel, Diane. "Betty Ford Center Fete Rates in Glitz, Glamour." *Los Angeles Times.* October 21, 1986, 2.

Roberts, Ants. "Fertiliser Industry—What Is Fertiliser?" *Te Ara—The Encyclopedia of New Zealand.* November 24, 2008, https://teara.govt.nz/en/fertiliser-industry/page-1.

Rodgers, Diana. "Eating Paleo Can Save the World" (blog). *Robb Wolf: Revolutionary Solutions to Modern Life,* January 13. 2013, https://robbwolf.com/2016/01/13/eating-paleo-can-save-the-world/.

Rosaldo, Renato. "From the Door of His Tent: The Fieldworker and the Inquisitor." In *Writing Culture: The Poetics and Politics of Ethnography*, edited by James Clifford and George Marcus, 91. Berkeley: University of California Press, 1986.

———. "Imperialist Nostalgia." *Representations* 26 (Spring 1989): 107–122.

Rubin, Jordan. *The Maker's Diet for Weight Loss: 16-Week Strategy for Burning Fat, Cleansing Toxins, and Living a Healthier Life!* Lake Mary, FL: Siolam Strang Company, 2009.

———. *The Maker's Diet Revolution: The 10 Day Diet to Lose Weight and Detoxify Your Body, Mind and Spirit*. Shippensburg, PA: Destiny Image Publishers, 2013.

———. *The Maker's Diet: The 40-Day Health Experience That Will Change Your Life Forever*. Shippensburg, PA: Destiny Image Publishers, 2004.

———. *Patient Heal Thyself: A Remarkable Health Program Combining Ancient Wisdom with Groundbreaking Clinical Research*. Topanga, CA: Freedom Press, 2003.

Russ, Kenneth. *The Palm Springs Diet: An Old Stone Age Diet for Modern Times*. Bloomington, IN: AuthorHouse, 2007.

Sagastume, Adolfo. *The Jesus Diet*. n.p. (eBook): Amazon Digital Services, 2011.

Saguy, Abigail. *What's Wrong with Fat?* New York: Oxford University Press, 2013.

Salisbury, James. *The Relation of Alimentation and Diseases*. New York: J. H. Vail and Co., 1888.

Saltus, Richard. "Some Scientists Skeptical of an Obesity Cure." *Boston Globe*. July 28, 1995, 3.

Sanborn, Geoffrey. *The Sign of the Cannibal: Melville and the Making of a Postcolonial Reader*. Durham, NC: Duke University Press, 1998.

Sands, Neil. "Pacific Nations Battle Obesity Epidemic." *The Independent*. April 11, 2011.

Santora, Marc. "Teenagers' Suit Says McDonald's Made Them Obese." *The New York Times*. November 21, 2002.

Sargent, Lyman Tower. "The Three Faces of Utopianism Revisited." *Utopian Studies* 5, no. 1 (1994): 1–37.

———. *Utopianism: A Very Short Introduction*. Oxford: Oxford University Press, 2010.

Satter, Beryl. *Each Mind a Kingdom: American Women, Sexual Purity, and the New Thought Movement, 1875–1920*. Berkeley: University of California Press, 1999.

Savard, Marie, with Carol Svec. *The Body Shape Solution to Weight Loss and Wellness: The Apples & Pears Approach to Losing Weight, Living Longer, and Feeling Healthier*. New York: Atria Books, 2001.

Schulz, Leslie, and Lisa Chaudhari. "High-Risk Populations: The Pimas of Arizona and Mexico." *Current Obesity Reports* 4, no. 1 (2015): 92–98.

Schwartz, David, and Hamilton Stapell. "Modern Cavemen? Stereotypes and Reality of the Ancestral Health Movement." *Journal of Evolution and Health* 1, no. 1 (2013): 2–10.

Schwartz, Hillel. *Never Satisfied: A Cultural History of Diets, Fantasies and Fat*. New York: Doubleday, 1986.

Schwartz, Robert M. *Holy Eating: The Spiritual Secret to Eternal Weight Loss*. Bloomington, IN: iUniverse, 2012.

Scrinis, Gyorgy. "On the Ideology of Nutritionism." *Gastronomica* 8, no. 1 (2008): 39–48.

Scrivner, Jane. "Clean Break." *The Times of India.* January 24, 1998, 1.

Seccombe, Mike. "Bum Deal on Back End of Big Birds." *The Global Mail.* November 19, 2013.

Selway, Oliver. *Instinctive Fitness.* St Albans, UK: Ecademy Press, 2012.

Shamblin, Gwen. *The Weigh Down Diet: Gwen Shamblin's Inspirational Way to Lose Weight, Stay Slim, and Find a New You.* New York: Doubleday, 1997.

Shedd, Charles. *The Fat Is in Your Head.* New York: Avon Books, 1972.

———. *Pray Your Weight Away.* Philadelphia: Lippincott, 1957.

Shefferman, Maurice. *Foods for Longer Living.* New York: Whittier Books, 1956.

Shintani, Terry. *The HawaiiDiet.* New York: Pocket Books, 1997.

Shintani, Terry, and Claire Ku'uleilani Hughes. *The Wai'anae Book of Hawaiian Health.* Wai'anae, HI: Wai'anae Coast Comprehensive Health Center, 1991.

Shintani, Terry, with Sheila Beckham, Helen Kanawaliwali O'Conner, Claire Ku'uleilani Hughes, and Alvin Sato. "The Waianae Diet Program: A Culturally Sensitive, Community-Based Obesity and Clinical Intervention Program for the Native Hawaiian Population." *Hawaiian Medical Journal* 53, no. 5 (May 1994): 136–141.

Siegel, Robert. "Samoans Await the Return of the Tasty Turkey Tail." *NPR: All Things Considered* (radio broadcast). May 9, 2013.

Singer, Merrill. "Following the Turkey Tails: Neoliberal Globalization and the Political Ecology of Health." *Journal of Political Ecology* 21 (2014): 436–451.

Sisson, Mark. *The Primal Blueprint: Reprogram Your Genes for Effortless Weight Loss, Vibrant Health, and Boundless Energy.* Malibu, CA: Primal Nutrition, 2012.

———. *The Primal Connection: Follow Your Genetic Blueprint to Health and Happiness.* Malibu, CA: Primal Nutrition, 2013.

Smith, Laura Harris. *The 30-Day Faith Detox: Renew Your Mind, Cleanse Your Body, Heal Your Spirit.* Bloomington, MN: Chosen Books, 2016.

Smith, Samuel Stanhope. *An Essay on the Causes of the Variety of Complexion and Figure in the Human Species.* New-Brunswick: NJ: J. Simpson and Co., 1810. In the Hathi Trust Digital Library, https://babel.hathitrust.org/cgi/pt?id=pst.000006225438.

"Society Beauties Seek Health & Complexion in Vegetables." *Chicago Daily Tribune.* July 23, 1905.

Somer, Elizabeth. *The Origin Diet: How Eating Like Our Stone Age Ancestors Will Maximize Your Health.* New York: Henry Holt, 2001.

Sonnen-Hernandez, Barbra. *The JESUS Diet: Taking the Weight off Your Soul.* n.p. (eBook): Zondervan, 2011.

Spark, Arlene, Lauren Dinour, and Janel Obenchain. *Nutrition in Public Health: Principles, Policies, and Practice.* Boca Raton, LA: CRC Press, 2007.

Squires, Nick. "Obesity Epidemic Destroying Paradise: South Pacific Crisis." *National Post.* February 22, 2007.

Stannard, David. "The Hawaiians: Health, Justice, and Sovereignty." *Cultural Survival Quarterly* 24, no. 1 (2000).

Stearns, Peter. *Fat History: Bodies and Beauty in the Modern West.* New York: New York University Press, 1997.

Stefansson, Vilhjalmur. *My Life with the Eskimo*. New York: The Macmillan Company, 1913.

Steinfeld, Henning. *Livestock's Long Shadow: Environmental Issues and Options*. Rome: Food and Agriculture Organization of the United Nations, 2006.

Stephenson, Nell. *Paleoista: Gain Energy, Get Lean and Feel Fabulous with the Diet You Were Born to Eat*. New York: Simon & Schuster, 2012.

Stiles, Anne. "The Rest Cure, 1873–1925." *BRANCH (Britain, Representation and Nineteenth-Century History)*. http://www.branchcollective.org/?ps_articles=anne-stiles-the-rest-cure-1873-1925.

Stone, Rachel Marie. *Eat with Joy: Redeeming God's Gift of Food*. Downers Grove, IL: Inter-Varsity Press, 2013.

Streitfeld, David. "Back to the Stone Age." *The Washington Post*. September 8, 1987.

Sturm, Roland, and Aiko Hattori. "Morbid Obesity Rates Continue to Rise Rapidly in the United States." *International Journal of Obesity* 37, no. 6 (June 2013): 889–891.

Sugar Research Foundation. *A Suggested Program for the Cane and Beet Sugar Industries*. October 1942, https://archive.org/details/480900-a-suggested-program-for-the-cane-and-beet-sugar.

"Suit in Fen-Phen Death Ends with Settlement." *Philadelphia Inquirer*. January 28, 2000.

Surface, Frank, and Raymond L. Bland. *American Food in the World War and Reconstruction Period: Operations of the Organizations under the Direction of Herbert Hoover, 1914 to 1924*. Stanford, CA: Stanford University Press, 1931.

Suvin, Darko. *Metamorphoses of Science Fiction: On the Poetics and History of a Literary Genre*. New Haven, CT: Yale University Press, 1979.

Tanner, Shannon. *Diets Don't Work . . . But Jesus Does!* Maitland, FL: Xulon Press, 2007.

Taylor, Kate. "Chipotle's Stock Is Down after Claims of Food-Poisoning Incidents in Manhattan." *Business Insider*. July 7, 2016, http://www.businessinsider.com/chipotles-stock-down-after-reports-of-another-food-poisoning-2016-7.

Taylor, Renée. *My Life on a Diet: Confessions of a Hollywood Diet Junkie*. New York: Putnam, 1986.

Teepen, Tom. "Commentary: Americans Live in 'Toxic Food Environment.'" *Dayton Daily News*. March 12, 2004, A10.

Telamon Press. *The Paleo Weight Loss Plan*. Berkeley, CA: Telamon Press, 2013.

TerKeurst, Lysa. *Made to Crave: Satisfying Your Deepest Desire with God, Not Food*. Grand Rapids, MI: Zondervan, 2011.

Teslenko, Tatiana. *Feminist Utopian Novels of the 1970s: Joanna Russ & Dorothy Bryant*. New York: Routledge, 2003.

Thompson, Vance. *Eat and Grow Thin: The Mahdah Menus*. New York: E. P. Dutton & Company, 1914.

Tompkins, Kyla Wazana. *Racial Indigestion: Eating Bodies in the 19th Century*. New York: New York University Press, 2012.

Tracy, Sarah W. *Alcoholism in America: From Reconstruction to Prohibition*. Baltimore: Johns Hopkins University Press, 2005.

Trask, Haunani-Kay. *From a Native Daughter: Colonialism, and Sovereignty in Hawai'i*. Monroe, ME: Common Courage Press, 1993.

Tukuitonga, Colin. "Pacific Island Health—Diseases and Disabilities." *Te Ara—The Encyclopedia of New Zealand*. July 13, 2012, https://teara.govt.nz/en/pacific-island-health/page-3.

United States Department of Agriculture. *Growth Patterns in the U.S. Organic Industry*. October 2013, http://www.ers.usda.gov/amber-waves/2013-october/growth-patterns-in-the-us-organic-industry.asp.

———. "USDA Reports Record Growth in U.S. Organic Producers" (press release). April 4, 2016, https://www.usda.gov/media/press-releases/2016/04/04/usda-reports-record-growth-us-organic-producers.

United States Department of Agriculture's Nutrition Evidence Library. *Scientific Report of the 2015 Dietary Guidelines Advisory Committee*, 8. https://health.gov/dietaryguidelines/2015-scientific-report/08-chapter-3/d3-7.asp.

United States Department of Health and Human Services, National Institute of Diabetes and Digestive and Kidney Diseases. *Overweight and Obesity Statistics*. October 2012, https://www.niddk.nih.gov/health-information/health-statistics/overweight-obesity.

Veit, Helen Zoe. *Modern Food, Moral Food: Self-Control, Science, and the Rise of Modern American Eating in the Early Twentieth Century*. Chapel Hill, NC: University of North Carolina Press, 2013.

Vertinsky, Patricia. "Embodying Normalcy: Anthropometry and the Long Arm of William H. Sheldon's Somatotyping Project." *Journal of Sport History* 29, no. 1 (Spring 2002): 95–133.

Vester, Katharina. "Regime Change: Gender, Class, and the Invention of Dieting in Post-Bellum America." *Journal of Social History* 44, no. 1 (Fall 2010): 39–70.

———. *A Taste of Power: Food and American Identities*. Berkeley: University of California Press, 2015.

Villepigue, James, and Rick Collins. *Alpha Male Challenge*. Emmaus, PA: Rodale Press, 2009.

Voegtlin, Walter. *The Stone Age Diet: Based on In-Depth Studies of Human Ecology and the Diet of Man*. New York: Vantage Press, 1975.

Warner, John. *Rousseau and the Problem of Human Relations*. University Park: Pennsylvania State University Press, 2015.

Warren, Rick, Daniel Amen, and Mark Hyman. *The Daniel Plan: 40 Days to a Healthier Life*. Grand Rapids, MI: Zondervan, 2013.

War-Time Cook and Health Book. In the John W. Hartman Center for Sales, Advertising & Marketing History, Rare Book, Manuscript, and Special Collections Library, Duke University.

Weaver, La Vita. *Fit for God: The 8-Week Plan That Kicks the Devil Out and Invites Health and Healing In*. New York: Doubleday, 2004.

Webb, Douglas. "Trading Health for Wealth? Obesity in the South Pacific." *United Nations Development Programme*. April 19, 2013, http://www.undp.org/content/undp/en/home/ourperspective/ourperspective-articles/2013/04/19/trading-health-for-wealth-obesity-in-the-south-pacific-doug-webb.html.

Wells, Spencer. *Pandora's Seed: Why the Hunter-Gatherer Holds the Key to Our Survival*. New York: Random House, 2011.

Wendt, Albert. "Towards a New Oceania." *Mana Review* 1 (1976): 49–60.

Wharton, Charles H. *Metabolic Man—Ten Thousand Years from Eden: The Long Search for a Personal Nutrition from our Forest Origins to the Supermarkets of Today.* Orlando, FL: Winmark Publishing, 2001.

White, Geoffrey, and Ty P. Kāwika Tengan. "Disappearing Worlds: Anthropology and Cultural Studies in Hawai'i and the Pacific." *Contemporary Pacific* 13, no. 2 (Fall 2001): 381–416.

Wild Man Foods. "Mission." *About Us.* March 11, 2014, http://www.wildmanfoods.org/mission.

Williams, Louise, and Peter Williams. "Evaluation of a Tool for Rating Popular Diet Books." *Nutrition and Dietetics* 60, no. 3 (2003): 185–197.

Willey, Angela. "Peters, Lulu Hunt." In *Diets and Dieting: A Cultural Encyclopedia*, edited by Sander Gilman, 211–212. New York: Routledge, 2008.

Williden, Mikki. "Primal Pacific: The Efficacy of a Culturally Appropriate LCHF Diet Trial for Reducing Health Risk among Pacific Employees." Paper presented at the Ancestral Health Symposium, Berkeley, CA, August 2014.

Wilson, Jacque. "Paleo Diet Ranks Last on 'Best Diets' List." *CNN.* January 7, 2014.

Wilson, Rob. "Introduction: Toward Imagining a New Pacific." In *Inside Out: Literature, Cultural Politics, and Identity in the New Pacific*, edited by Vilsoni Hereniko and Rob Wilson. Oxford: Rowman and Littlefield, 1999.

Winters, Joseph. "Toward an Embodied Utopia: Marcuse, The Re-Ordering of Desire, and the 'Broken' Promise of Post-Liberal Practices." *Telos*, no. 165 (Winter 2013): 151–168.

Wolf, Bryan. *Romantic Re-Vision: Culture and Consciousness in Nineteenth-Century American Painting and Literature.* Chicago: University of Chicago Press, 1982.

Wolf, Naomi. *The Beauty Myth: How Images of Beauty Are Used against Women.* New York: W. Morrow, 1991.

Wolf, Robb. *The Paleo Solution: The Original Human Diet.* Las Vegas, NV: Victory Belt, 2010.

Wolfe, Alexandra. "Pastor Rick Warren: Fighting Obesity with Faith." *The Wall Street Journal.* January 17, 2014.

Womble, Leslie, and Thomas Wadden. "Commercial and Self-Help Weight Loss Programs." In *Eating Disorders and Obesity: A Comprehensive Handbook*, edited by Christopher G. Fairburn and Kelly D. Brownell. New York: Guilford Press, 2002.

World Health Organization. *Obesity: Preventing and Managing the Global Epidemic.* Geneva: WHO, 1998.

Yager, Susan. *The Hundred Year Diet: America's Voracious Appetite for Losing Weight.* Emmaus, PA: Rodale Press, 2010.

Zallinger, Rudolph. "The Road to Homo Sapiens." Illustration in F. Clark Howell, *Early Man.* New York: Time-Life Books, 1965.

Zellerbach, Merla, with Phyllis Saifer. *Detox: A Successful & Supportive Program for Freeing Your Body from the Physical and Psychological Effects of Chemical Pollutants at Home & at Work, Junk Food Additives, Sugar, Nicotine, Drugs, Alcohol, Caffeine, Prescription and Non-prescription Medications, and Other Environmental Toxins.* Los Angeles: J. P. Tarcher, 1984.

Zimmet, Paul. "Epidemiology of Diabetes and Its Macrovascular Manifestations in Pacific Populations: The Medical Effects of Social Progress." *Diabetes Care* 2, no. 2 (March 1979): 144–145.

————. "Globalization, Coca-Colonization and the Chronic Disease Epidemic: Can the Doomsday Scenario Be Averted?" *Journal of Internal Medicine* 247, no. 3 (2000): 309.

Zimmet, Paul, with Gary Dowse and Caroline Finch. "The Epidemiology and Natural History of NIDDM—Lessons from the South Pacific." *Diabetes/Metabolism Research and Reviews* 6 (1990): 91–124.

Zubkovs, Jani. *Why Women Love Cavemen—A Man's Guide to Tame the Bitch.* New York: Bonnie's Gang, 2009.

Zuk, Marlene. *Paleofantasy: What Evolution Really Tells Us about Sex, Diet, and How We Live.* New York: W. W. Norton, 2013.

INDEX

ABOUT THE AUTHOR

ADRIENNE ROSE BITAR is a postdoctoral associate in the History department at Cornell University. She is a cultural historian whose research and teaching focuses on food studies and the medical humanities. Previous research publications include work on competitive eating, couponing, the Paleo diet, locavorism, and the history of the American West. She received her Modern Thought and Literature PhD from Stanford University in 2016.